THE WORLD'S MOST
SENSATIONAL
SEX LIVES

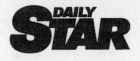

THE WORLD'S MOST
SENSATIONAL
SEX LIVES

BY
NIGEL BLUNDELL

SUNBURST BOOKS

PHOTOGRAPHY CREDITS

Express Newspapers Plc: 64, 126, 131, 135, 146, 156, 169.
Mary Evans Picture Library: 21, 29.
Rex Pictures: 89:
USA New York: 115.
London Features International: 121.
George Phillips: 175.
Maxwell Picture Agency: 180.
News and Features New York: 184.
Frank Spooner Pictures: 189.
Copyright unknown: 52, 61, 161.

This edition published 1995 by Sunburst Books, Deacon House,
65 Old Church Street, London SW3 5BS

ISBN 1 85778 079 5

Printed and bound in the United Kingdom

Contents

Introduction

From the bedroom to the boardroom, men and women who should know better show themselves at their very worst.

Politicians, businessmen, movie stars, rock singers and royals ... all have been ready to risk every shred of respectability for a red-hot romance, a sensual soirée or a short-lived fling.

Yet they all knew what they were doing. They were all adults. They all knew the dreadful risks and the shame of exposure. So why did they persist in doing it?

The answer, of course, is SEX.

This three-letter word is responsible for the downfall of so many public figures. *The World's Most Sensational Sex Lives* charts the indiscretions of those who risked all for 'love'. Their stories are riveting tales of deceit and intrigue, but ultimately, all end in exposure ...

QUEEN CAROLINE

Royal marriages in Britain are steeped in a long tradition of cant, hypocrisy, and scandal. But few come close to the disastrous match between the pompous, spendthrift, unpopular George IV and the unattractive Caroline of Brunswick.

The reasons why George decided to get married are obvious. He needed help in reducing his staggering £630,000 debts, which the British Parliament had pointedly refused to clear. A deal was struck in which the necessary funds would be found, as long as George, then Prince of Wales, married and produced an heir.

The fact that the Prince chose to march down the aisle with Caroline in April 1795, rather than the beautiful, intelligent Louise of Mecklenburg-Strelitz, can only be guessed at. One theory is that his mistress at the time, Lady Jersey, regarded Caroline as less of a sexual rival and managed to influence George's decision. Her judgement was spot on.

When George was introduced to Caroline at St James's Palace he was dumbstruck. He liked nothing about her. Falling into a pit of depression, he began drinking heavily.

The honeymoon, on which Lady Jersey was a

guest, was a farce. George shied away from his bride at every opportunity although, mindful of his bargain with Parliament, he did consummate the marriage. Caroline was pregnant within a few months. Meanwhile, the 'proud' father-to-be continued to treat her like an outcast.

A year later he wrote to her in an attempt to explain why he didn't want to continue their sexual relationship. "Our inclinations are not in our power," he pleaded, adding that being 'polite' most certainly was. Caroline was baffled and asked her friend, the politician George Canning, what the letter meant. Canning told her she had licence to do whatever she wished as long as she was discreet. Eagerly, she embarked on a torrid affair with him.

Caroline now moved to her own home in Blackheath, South East London. Soon the first rumours began to emerge of her sexual notoriety; a four-year-old boy in the house, William Austin, was said to be her illegitimate son. This sparked what became known at Court as the 'Delicate Investigation'. Caroline was cleared of impropriety, though she later claimed the child was hers by Prince Louis Ferdinand of Prussia, her first love.

In August 1814 Caroline left England to settle in Naples, where she became the mistress of Napoleon's brother-in-law King Joachim. She moved on just as Napoleon was escaping from Elba, and travelled to Munich, Athens, Constantinople, Tunis and Jerusalem with one of the former Emperor's couriers, Italian Bartolomeo Bergami. Together they acted for all the world like man and wife.

In 1820, George III died after suffering years of insanity. George IV was the new king, which meant Caroline was now Queen of England. She rejected the government's offer of a £50,000 no-questions-asked cash payment to stay abroad and hurried back to claim her rightful place. Desperate to prevent her attending the coronation, Lord Liverpool's government hauled her before the House of Lords on a charge of 'a most unbecoming and degrading intimacy with a foreigner of low station' (Bergami). The aim was to get the king the divorce he desired.

To her surprise, the queen enlisted massive support from the public. George IV was loathed in every corner of his kingdom and consequently she found her coach escorted by a cheering throng every time she attended Parliament. Confronted by hostility, the Lords' abandoned their divorce bill.

Lord Liverpool banned Caroline from attending the coronation, set for 29 April 1821, but it made no difference. She arrived dressed in a muslin outfit and screamed through the doors of

Westminster Abbey: "The queen – open." The pages on duty did her bidding, but as she roared "I am the Queen of England," a courtier cried to the guard: "Do your duty. Shut the hall door." It was slammed in her face.

Caroline died two weeks later amid wide rumours that she had been poisoned. George IV lived for a further nine years. His subjects seemed to regard his dying as the most noble thing he ever did.

LORD BYRON

From the moment he was introduced to lovemaking by a nymphomaniac servant girl at the age of nine, Lord Byron found himself drawn to the wilder side of sex.

The girl, Mary Gray, would undress before his transfixed gaze or perform intercourse with her numerous boyfriends in front of him. The experience seems to have fuelled his belief that he was attractive to women and probably convinced him that sex was nothing without variation and experimentation.

And so he embarked on a quest to satisfy his sexual urges: a quest that led him to the beds of more than 200 prostitutes, saw him commit incest with his half-sister and father her child, sodomise his wife, and indulge his taste for young boys at every opportunity.

His personal life became a tempestuous sex scandal that transformed him from the darling of Regency London into a society demon. Ultimately, it turned him into a pathetic creature who died a lonely and embittered outcast.

Born George Gordon on 28 January 1788, Byron hardly knew his father. It was probably just as well. 'Mad Jack' was a waster and womaniser who had already had one adulterous affair (with the Marchioness of Carmarthen). Byron's mother, Catherine Gordon, was an unprepossessing Scots heiress who spent almost her entire £23,000 fortune on sustaining Jack's outrageous lifestyle. The birth of little George seems to have been a watershed in the marriage. Soon afterwards, Mad Jack deserted his family to begin a new life in France and died three years later.

At school George was teased mercilessly because of his deformed right foot. He got little solace at home, where his mother would sometimes refer to him as 'that lame brat'. Her tantrums and violent mood swings probably planted the seeds of his distrust of women. Increasingly he escaped from the harsh realities of life into his books, especially historical accounts and stories set in the Mediterranean.

At ten he inherited the title of Lord Byron with the death of his grandfather and moved to Newstead Abbey, Nottingham, a crumbling pile which could have been designed straight from the imagination of a romantic poet. He began his first term at Harrow School and almost certainly had his first experience of homosexuality there. Later, in his teens, he found himself simultaneously in love with both his cousin, Mary Parker, and a neighbour, Mary Chaworth.

It was not until 1805, however, that his sexual appetite truly emerged. At Cambridge he spent many an evening with prostitutes, at least one of whom claimed he was too rough as a lover.

About this time he also re-acquainted himself with his half-sister Augusta, then married to a Colonel George Leigh, and fell for a choirboy called Edleston. He always insisted his relationship with the latter was 'pure', itself a tacit admission that friendships with other boys were not. In his last months at Cambridge he seduced his first mistress, a woman named Caroline, who willingly accommodated his desires by dressing up as a boy.

At 21, Byron left England for a grand tour of the Mediterranean. His first published poems had not been well received and he may have felt in need of some inspiration. The trip also allowed him to expand his sexual experience. In between regular visits to prostitutes, he would entertain a fifteen-year-old Greek boy called Nicolo.

Byron later recalled how he once came upon a cart which carried a jumping, wriggling sack. Bribing the driver to cut it open, he was shown a woman awaiting execution for being unfaithful to her husband. The poet immediately recognised her as a prostitute of his acquaintance and, his protective instincts aroused, managed to save her from being cast into the sea.

Returning to England in 1812, Byron found himself with a newly acquired status. His poem,

Childe Harold's Pilgrimage, about a young man jaded by over-indulgence in forbidden pastimes, was hugely popular and turned him into something of a sex symbol. It reached the point where some fashionable young men would try to copy his sullen stares, moody silences, even his limp!

One of his female admirers was Lady Caroline Lamb, wife of the politician William Lamb. She would later describe him as 'mad, bad and dangerous to know' but it seems that, for a time at least, she was obsessively in love with him. In one attempt to grab his attention she even dressed herself up as a pageboy and hid in his coach. For a while he found her pranks amusing but later he grew bored with them. He also disliked her overt sexuality and when she sent him one of her pubic hairs as a love token it was the beginning of the end of their relationship.

Soon afterwards he fled into the arms of his half-sister Augusta, as much for the prospect of committing incest as for any deep love between them. He also paid visits to the sex-mad Lady Oxford, all the while continuing to fend off the persistent Caroline Lamb.

Gossip about his private life was juicily savoured by London society. In an attempt to quieten the rumours Byron opted for respectability and the quiet life by marrying a rather dull heiress called Annabella Milbanke. Their first days of marriage together were rather tainted by the poet's assertion that he was bound on principal to hate anyone he wed. However, he soon found that marriage suited him rather better than he had expected.

This was no doubt in part due to Annabella's complete innocence about matters sexual. Byron convinced her that by subjecting herself to sodomy she was merely fulfilling a normal variation of sex with which any dutiful wife would be happy to comply. This state of affairs continued until after Annabella bore him a daughter and took the child to her parents, Sir Ralph and Lady Milbanke, to recuperate.

Annabella talked openly of the act of sodomy, a revelation which must have caused her poor mother to almost choke on her wine. The Milbankes had conservative views about sex and made it clear to their daughter that she would not be returning to a man whose marital perversions were undoubtably a criminal offence.

The collapse of the marriage turned Byron into one of the most despised men in Regency England. This was in part due to the 'British disease' of toppling public figures trapped in scandal, but was also the result of outrageous indiscretions by the poet and some of his wealthy lovers. A man who relished the criminal acts of sodomy and incest hardly made himself popular as a party guest.

Byron responded to such pointed snubs the only way he knew how. He resolved to leave England. But first he ordered himself a magnificent new £500 coach and embarked upon one last, passionate affair with a girl called Claire Clairemont.

This single night of lovemaking left Claire pregnant and caused Byron's close friend, the poet Shelley, to remonstrate with him for ravishing such a nubile young woman. With a typically self-centred response, Byron retorted that "no one has been more carried off than poor dear me."

By 1818 he was lodging with a draper in Venice and wasted no time in seducing his hapless host's wife, Marianna. They regularly made love three times a day until he fell for an attractive peasant girl, Margarita Cogni, and then a married woman barely out of a convent, Teresa Guiccioli. When the sale of his Newstead mansion netted £94,500 he quickly diverted the proceeds into a rented palazzo, a house that became his personal brothel.

Inevitably, Byron's tangled love life caught up with him. Teresa left her aging husband and tried to convert him to a life of domesticity. His misery at this prospect was combined with sadness at the deaths of his daughter Allegra – conceived with Claire Clairemont – and his friend Shelley. Byron packed his bags and moved to Greece. It was there he died of a fever, aged only 37, alone, bored and, perhaps, longing for home.

Sadly, the story of Byron's life through his own words will never be known. After he died his friends Tom Moore and John Hobhouse met his publisher John Murray to make a decision on the poet's memoirs. Moore wanted to keep them for posterity. Hobhouse and Murray could not agree. They were appalled by the sexual behaviour described and insisted the whole bundle was thrown on the office fire. Had they retained the manuscript, it would almost certainly have become Byron's biggest seller.

OSCAR WILDE

I'll be famous, and if not famous, I'll be notorious – those words, penned by Oscar Wilde in a letter during his last year at university in Oxford, turned out to be unerringly accurate.

His entire life was a curious mixture of fame and notoriety. Many of those who admired his literary genius could not help but loathe his sexual activities.

As a child, Wilde was given a first-hand glimpse of the mechanism that would be his future downfall: a libel battle. His mother, Lady Jane, was sued by a young woman called Mary Travers, who claimed Jane had unjustly labelled her a blackmailer. Though Travers eventually won a mere farthing in damages, the Wildes were ordered to pay all legal costs.

The judgement was a huge financial blow to the family. Yet the memory of it failed to deter Oscar when in later life he issued his fateful writ through the High Court in London.

Wilde's rich literary talent first began to shine in 1871 when, aged seventeen, he won a scholarship to Dublin's Trinity College. Under his mentor, Professor of Ancient History the Reverend John Pentland Mahaffy, he discovered

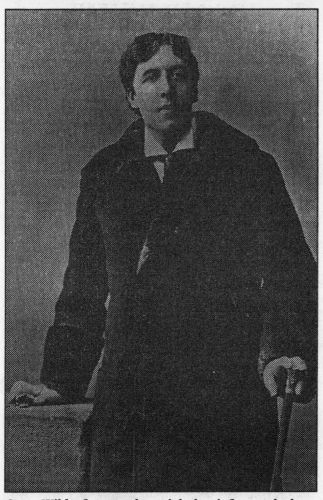

Oscar Wilde: famous playwright but infamous lecher.

a love of the classics, particularly all things Greek. It was there he learnt of the Mediterranean tradition of pederasty. He was fascinated and, though still heterosexual by inclination, he began to ponder what it would be like to take a boy lover.

At Oxford he was guided through the intricacies of classical art and architecture by the likes of John Ruskin and Walter Pater. Pater's conviction that life should be enjoyed with 'gem-like flame' was one of the cornerstones of Wilde's own philosophy. Already he was reaching the conclusion that beauty was the ultimate value.

His first published poems coincided with his arrival in media circles in London. He met Lillie Langtry, the Prince of Wales's mistress, and promptly fell in love with her. He also began cocking a snook at the accepted social norms of fashionable London. Announcing that a revolution in dress was more important than a revolution in morals, he paraded around the West End sporting a knee-length velvet coat edged in braid, black silk stockings and knee breeches.

If nothing else it produced great publicity. By the early 1880s the satirical magazine *Punch* was running a number of scathing send-ups of Wilde, while another well-known publication, *Patience*, depicted him in the fictional guise of a negligibly-talented poet called Bunthorne.

If *Patience* hoped to irritate Wilde, however, the strategy failed dismally. He lapped up the extra publicity and believed it led directly to an invitation for him to perform a US lecture tour.

The tour kicked off in New York where Wilde, arriving at port immigration, uttered the words which became his unofficial epitaph: "I have nothing to declare but my genius."

Though his visit was a success, he had little time for the love affair between the Irish and the Americans. He later commented dryly: "Of course, if one had enough money to go to America, one wouldn't go."

Back in England in 1883 Wilde became engaged to Constance Lloyd, a woman he loved passionately and who later bore him two sons. But the marriage faltered when, two years later, he discovered he still had traces of syphilis (caught from an Oxford prostitute) in his bloodstream. The so-called 'mercury cure' he had taken had failed to expunge the disease and he reluctantly decided to end sexual relations with Constance.

His concern did not, however, extend to the welfare of his first gay lover, a seventeen-year-old boy called Robbie Ross. In fairness to Wilde, this may have been because he did not indulge in sodomy. It appears from his own confessions to friends that his taste in homosexual activity was mainly for fondling and mutual masturbation while sitting the chosen boy on his knee.

He also avoided overtly feminine youths, preferring masculine 'rough trade'. He described sex with these coarse types as "like dining with panthers," and once admitted having five telegraph messenger boys in a single night. Each had kisses planted all over his body and Oscar later admitted candidly: "They were all dirty and appealed to me for that reason."

Over the next few years Wilde gradually built up a literary reputation as a writer of plays, short stories and magazine articles. But in 1891 the notoriety he had predicted in his student days abruptly arrived with the publication of *The Picture of Dorian Gray*, which relishingly told the story of a young rake's descent into the vilest fleshpots of vice-ridden London.

About the same time he began a sexual relationship with Lord Alfred Douglas, son of the Marquess of Queensbury.

The marquess remains best known for his development of the laws of boxing, the so-called Queensbury rules. But his other claim to fame centres on his role in the downfall of Oscar Wilde.

In 1893 Lord Douglas passed on an old suit to a jobless young clerk who was a casual friend. In one pocket the youth found a love letter from

Wilde, which he promptly use to try to extort money.

He might as well have tried to cut cheese off the moon. Wilde scathingly informed him that the letter could be interpreted in different ways and that "art is rarely intelligible to the criminal classes." The persistent blackmailer replied that he could get £60 for the letter. But he was quite unprepared for Wilde's advice to strike the deal immediately. Deciding that crime didn't pay after all, the hard-up clerk handed back the note.

Unfortunately for Wilde, a copy had already found its way to the Marquess of Queensbury who was incandescent with rage at the phrase: "It is a marvel that those rose-red lips of yours should have been made no less for music of song than for the madness of kisses."

The marquess, an eccentric Scot prone to temper tantrums, forbade his son from ever meeting Wilde again (an order derided by Alfred). He also boasted loudly of his intention to introduce the poet to a fist fight, and took to following him around his London haunts.

The feud came to a head when the marquess called at Wilde's club, the Albemarle, and presented his calling card at the door. The note written on it read: "To Oscar Wilde, posing as a somdomite(sic)." When Wilde received it he was quick to see an opportunity for revenge.

He engaged his solicitor Charles Humphries to draw up a libel tort and brought the case on the grounds that he had never committed the criminal offence of sodomy.

Wilde's claim was probably true but the business of sueing involves much more than the pursuit of truth. English libel laws are concerned with protecting an individual's reputation in the eyes of 'right-thinking members of society generally'. If a wronged individual already has a dubious reputation then his chances in court are often slim.

Wilde's case was doomed from the moment defence lawyers threatened to expose his encounters with boys at London's Savoy Hotel. Suddenly, rather than the wronged man, he was the man on trial.

On the very day the marquess was acquitted of the libel charge police obtained a warrant for Wilde's arrest, and on 6 April 1895 he was put on trial charged with committing acts of indecency.

The jury failed to reach a verdict and the judge ordered a retrial. The second trial, at which a succession of Wilde's young male lovers told how they had submitted to sodomy, oral sex and masturbation, ended with a guilty verdict. Wilde was sentenced to two years' hard labour, an experience he later recounted so poignantly in his poem *The Ballad of Reading Gaol*.

On his release in May 1897, Wilde realised he had changed. His passion for writing had gone; "something is killed in me," was the way he put it.

He became an exile in Paris under the name Sebastian Melmoth, taken from Maturin's Gothic story *Melmoth the Wanderer*. On 30 November 1900 he died penniless in a downmarket hotel.

LILLIE LANGTRY AND EDWARD, PRINCE OF WALES

The love of Edward, Prince of Wales, for actress Lillie Langtry became the most talked-about, fascinating and scandalous affair of the era. By the time it had ended, the British Royal Family – and indeed Britain itself – would never be the same again.

Lillie, the pretty lass who would become the most shocking 'scarlet woman' of her time, was born on 13 October 1853 in Jersey, Channel Islands, as Emilie Charlotte Le Breton, the only sister among six brothers. Her father, the Dean of Jersey, was known by islanders as the 'Dirty Dean' because of his many affairs – and had to break up Lillie and one of her first teenage lovers because the boyfriend was one of his own illegitimate children.

Lillie learned from living in a predominantly male household how she could make it in a man's world. She may also have picked up her own passionate nature from her father. Indeed, she once referred to him as "a damned nuisance ... he couldn't be trusted with any woman anywhere."

The staid island of Jersey could not hold Lillie

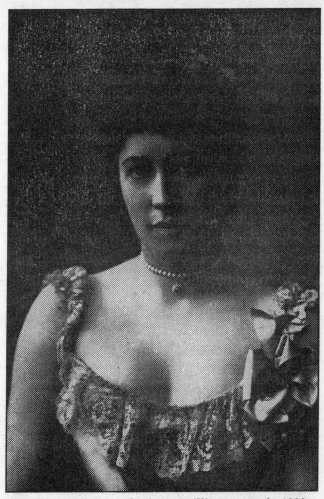

The 'Jersey Lily': royal mistress Lillie Langtry in 1890.

for long. In March 1874 she married 26-year-old Edward Langtry, the son of a wealthy Irish shipowner, who had berthed his 60ft yacht on the island. "To become the mistress of the yacht, I married the owner," she later admitted. Within a year she had persuaded her hapless husband to move to London, where she set about breaking into society.

She arrived in the capital as a stunning beauty, with a full figure, long, cascading hair, a flawless complexion and deep blue eyes. Overawed by the glamour and glitter of society, she came to realise that her beauty could be her ticket to freedom. She sought and accepted every invitation to every dinner party and soiree open to her.

At one such party she met the renowned portrait painter George Francis Miles who asked her to pose for him. Lillie agreed and before long she was gracing cards that sold for a penny apiece. Miles made a mint from them – and gave the reason thus: "She happens to be the most beautiful woman on earth."

One of those who asked to see the original portrait was Prince Edward, known to his friends as Bertie, to his detractors as Edward The Caresser, and later as King Edward VII. Having seen the portrait, he now yearned to see the flesh. He asked one of his cronies to effect an introduction. So, on 24 May 1877, the prince was invited to a dinner party thrown by his bachelor friend Sir Allen Young, who had also invited Lillie.

As the introductions were being made – and as Lillie's fawning husband was bowing his head with great regularity – the prince realised that here was a woman he had to possess. Lillie was only too willing, and they wasted no time.

During dinner, the prince leaned across to her and remarked that the artist had not done her justice; "her beauty," he said, "was even greater in person than it was in the portrait." She murmured her polite thanks but she knew from that moment that she had him hooked.

Within a week they were lovers. But this affair was to be different for the prince, who was no stranger to romantic liaisons with married women. In many of his previous liaisons, Edward had been relatively circumspect. During that age, many aristocrats kept mistresses but they were never flaunted in public; they were always kept at a discreet distance. Edward himself already had a wife, Princess Alexandra, and six children. He was the product of his mother Queen Victoria's moralistic age which disapproved of infidelities. Bertie suddenly viewed all this as hypocrisy – and determined to display his beautiful, new conquest to the world.

Edward built Lillie a house in Bournemouth

which they used as their weekend lovenest. He took her to sporting events, social functions, dinner parties and on numerous trips to Paris. Neither he nor she cared who saw them on these romantic forays to France and once, in full view of the elite dinner crowd at Maxim's restaurant, they brazenly and passionately kissed full on the lips. Back in England, however, they were slightly more discreet. At social gatherings such as Royal Ascot, they kept a distance. He would be accompanied by the long-suffering Princess Alexandra, while Lillie would be on the arm of her husband.

Eventually, however, Edward had had all he could take of this intrigue and he began demanding of his courtiers that his 'Jersey Lillie' be recognised by society as his 'official' mistress. So for three years they quite openly continued their torrid affair, thumbing their noses at the prudes who tut-tutted behind their backs. Whenever Bertie was invited to a party or ball, he would write Lillie's name on the RSVP and bring her along.

Lillie herself was in seventh heaven. She wrote at the time: "Each successive season brought with it the same orgy of convivial gatherings, balls, dinners, receptions, concerts, operas, etc., which at first seemed to me a dream, a delight, a wild excitement, and I concentrated on the pursuit of amusement with the wholeheartedness that is characteristic of me, flying from one diversion to another, from dawn to dawn."

Lillie saw as proof of her 'seal of approval' the fact that her royal lover actually introduced her to his mother, Queen Victoria, who was definitely not amused! Astonishingly, he also introduced Lillie to his wife, who could only bite her tongue and pretend to be ignorant of her husband's infidelities. But while Princess Alexandra handled the scandalous behaviour with royal aplomb, the cuckolded Edward Langtry could not. He sank into a life of alcoholism and heavy debt, while his wife was paraded around the the favourite haunts of European aristocracy.

Admiring crowds followed her through the streets, and everything she wore became an instant fashion trend. Even the colour of a dress could start a fad. Once she wore a pink dress to Ascot, and soon every high-class store in London featured that particular shade in the windows.

Unfortunately for Lillie, however, Edward's eye continued to rove. He became infatuated with French actress Sarah Bernhardt and tried to find another suitor for Lillie. After a while, he believed that he had successfully passed Lillie on to his nephew: a handsome naval officer named Prince Louis of Battenberg, who was to become the father of Lord Louis Mountbatten. The truth, however, was that Lillie was almost certainly already having an affair with the Battenberg prince long before she was dropped by Bertie!

Lillie's affair with Prince Louis also ended before long. She became pregnant with his child and he cruelly packed her off to France to have the baby in secret. She gave birth to a daughter, Jeanne-Marie, whom she passed off as her niece.

Lillie returned to Britain and in 1881, thanks to Prince Edward who had remained a friend, she fulfilled her ambition of entering the acting profession. She made her debut at the Haymarket Theatre in the role of Kate Hardcastle in *She Stoops To Conquer*, watched by the admiring prince and most of the social elite. She was again the toast of the town. Songs were written about her and her theatrical appearances were sell-outs.

She sailed to America where she gained a new army of admirers, playing New York to rapturous audiences. When in 1882 her luxuriously appointed rail coach visited Vinegaroon, Texas, the infamous 'hanging Judge' Roy Bean was so smitten that he changed the name of the town to Langtry in her honour. Lillie was by now a world celebrity, acclaimed as the most prestigious actress of her age.

There were, of course, further affairs. One of her lovers was even rumoured to have been the crusty, Bible-thumping British Prime Minister,

William Gladstone. In 1885, however, she at last found the great love that she had been searching for so long ...

Wealthy baronet Hugo de Bathe was the man, a healthy fifteen years her junior. They became lovers until 1897 when, upon the death of her husband in an asylum, Lillie was free to wed again. They moved to Monte Carlo where they lived in peace and harmony.

In 1901 Queen Victoria died and Bertie became king. But his reign was short. He died of a heart attack in 1910, due to his lifelong overindulgence. Lillie went to the funeral, then returned to Jersey to watch from a distance as the golden age of empire gave way to World War I.

In 1929 she died, aged 76. She was buried in St Saviour's churchyard, Jersey, not far from where she was born and close to where she had once, as a teenager, run naked through the island lanes to scandalise the local lads.

KITTY O'SHEA AND CHARLES PARNELL

It was an unlikely meeting that led Charles Parnell down the rocky road of a political sex scandal. He was leader of the Irish Party. Kitty O'Shea was the wife of one of his MPs. When their eyes met there was an instant infatuation.

That first meeting took place outside the House of Commons in 1880. For months Kitty had been writing to Parnell, inviting him to attend a series of dinner parties she was hosting at London's St Thomas's Hotel. The aim of these gatherings was to provide her husband Willie, the member for County Clare, with some influential political connections. Why, she now asked Parnell, could he not bring himself to turn up?

Later she recalled the confrontation in her autobiography. "He came out; a tall, gaunt figure, thin and deadly pale," she wrote. "He looked straight at me, smiling, and his curiously burning eyes looked into mine with a wonderful intentness that threw into my brain the sudden thought: 'This man is wonderful – and different.'"

"I asked him why he had not answered my last invitation to dinner, and if nothing would induce him to come. He answered that he had not opened his letters for days but, that if I would let him, he would come to dinner directly he returned from Paris."

"In leaning forward in the cab to say goodbye, a rose I was wearing in my bodice fell out onto my skirt. He picked it up and, touching it lightly with his lips, placed it in his buttonhole."

Kitty's colourful (and perhaps embroidered) account doesn't fully explain the complex reasons behind the love-at-first-sight affair. For a start, her marriage to Willie was in deep trouble. She had volunteered to help him improve his contacts partly out of a sense of duty, partly because she thought it might revive his disastrous business career and partly because she was fascinated by politicians.

Parnell on the other hand saw in her some of the characteristics he had loved so much in his mother. Her bubbling chatter, bold opinions and air of determination captivated him as no other woman had in years. He had noted that she was short and a little plump, but his lingering memory was of her beautiful hair.

Parnell had remained celibate since 1865, the year he ended a romance with a pretty, young, farmer's daughter back home in Avondale, County Wicklow. Then aged nineteen, he ditched the girl only to discover that she had committed suicide. His sister Fanny later claimed that he had been out in his boat when he saw her body fished out of the river. The experience left him devastated and for years afterwards he would suffer occasional fits of severe depression.

Parnell entered Parliament in 1875 as a committed proponent of Home Rule for Ireland. He soon realised the House of Commons would never accept the logic and reason behind his arguments so he and his supporters resolved to make as much of a nuisance of themselves as possible. They hoped mainland MPs would weary of these tactics and pack them off to Dublin to sit in their own Parliament.

One method adopted by the Home Rulers was to try and talk out proposed legislation, a technique known as filibustering. They would force the Commons into all-night sittings, sometimes holding up proceedings by as much as 26 hours with their continuous speeches. But Parnell was also prepared to court outright controversy where he deemed it necessary.

On 30 June 1876, after three Fenians (republican rebels) had been executed for allegedly murdering a policeman in Manchester, he boldly told the House of Commons that neither he nor anyone in Ireland would regard the three as anything other than martyrs.

His words made him an instant hero among

Fenians and his advocacy three years later of a rent strike by Irish tenants propelled him further into the political limelight. He was fast becoming Ireland's unofficial leader.

It was amid these mounting pressures that Parnell turned to Kitty O'Shea for solace and sex. On 22 September 1880 he spelt out his love for her in a letter from Dublin. "I cannot keep myself away from you any longer, so shall leave for London tonight," he wrote.

By now Parnell's health was poor and Willie O'Shea was quick to invite his leader to stay at his home in Eltham, London. Thrown together under the same roof, Kitty and Charles's affair secretly blossomed.

When he stood accused of 'conspiracy to impoverish landlords' it was she who suggested he hide in the dressing room adjoining her bedroom, bringing him his meals personally so that none of the servants would guess what was happening. It was a huge risk for a married Victorian woman to take, yet she accepted it almost with relish.

Even when he was free of the courts, Parnell's double-life continued to make huge demands on his mental reserves. He would write to Kitty in code, rent houses where they could meet freely under aliases and even resorted to twisting a handkerchief during Commons speeches as a sign that Kitty and he should meet later.

Willie, by now, was resigned to his sham marriage. He had guessed what was going on between his wife and Parnell but was prepared to accommodate the affair as long as it was conducted with maximum discretion.

It was only when he discovered Parnell's travelling trunk in a bedroom that he saw red and challenged the politician to a duel. Parnell handled himself with typical aplomb. It was vital, he argued, that Katharine acted as his medium in communications between the Home Rulers and Prime Minister Gladstone's government. Willie allowed himself to be persuaded.

On several occasions Kitty found herself pregnant. Her first daughter, born in February 1882, was registered in Willie's name, although Parnell was almost certainly the father. The child died within weeks but over the next three years Kitty gave birth to two more daughters, Clare and Katie, again registering them as the offspring of her husband. The tactic calmed Willie's fears and Parnell made sure he played a high-profile role in the talks between the Home Rulers and Gladstone. It was vital that the wronged husband be satisfied with his political lot.

As the festive season approached in 1889, talks over the Irish Question seemed close to fruition. Then, out of the blue, Willie O'Shea chose Christmas Eve to file for divorce. Perhaps he felt he was being ridiculed by an affair which was common knowledge among Westminster's gossip mongers. Perhaps he had simply had enough of the pretence. Whatever the reason his actions brought a viperous response from Kitty. Her counter-petition read:

"Years of neglect, varied by quarrels, had killed my love for him long before I met Parnell, and since February 1882 I could not bear to be near him."

The scandal, now forced into the open, left Parnell politically vulnerable. Gladstone made clear that if Home Rule talks were to continue it would be advisable for the Irishman to resign. Even Parnell's closest ally, John Redmond, admitted that in that event Gladstone would be the Home Ruler's natural leader because "he is the master of the party."

To which Parnell's principal rival Tim Healy scathingly replied: "Who is to be the mistress of the party?"

Stubbornly, Parnell refused to step down and succeeded in rallying his party around him. But the scandal had fatally wounded him in the eyes of Gladstone, Parliament and the British press. Talks on Home Rule reached stalemate and there is little doubt that the scandal delayed republican ambitions by 30 years. Neither did Kitty escape retribution. The magazine *Vanity Fair* referred to her as 'O'Shea Who Must Be Obeyed'.

Parnell and Kitty married in 1891, soon after her divorce was finalised. But their marriage lasted only a few months before he succumbed to his persistent poor health.

Kitty, drained by events of the past few years suffered a breakdown. She lived a further 30 years in relative anonymity.

REVEREND HAROLD DAVIDSON

At the turn of the last century the quiet English village of Stiffkey, Norfolk, was a picturesque though otherwise unremarkable paradigm of rural life. It was the kind of place where locals joked to each other about nothing ever happening; where the only chance for a gossip was at the public house or the church, and where the word 'scandal' simply did not rear its ugly head.

Until, that is, the Reverend Harold Francis Davidson walked onto the scene.

His entire life was a tabloid newspaperman's dream, a whoring clergyman caught on film with naked schoolgirls and who ended his days being mauled and eaten by a lion. Yet there is another side to Davidson, a side which suggests he suffered from some kind of mental disorder which saddled him with multiple personalities. Whatever the truth, he is certainly one of the strangest men ever to slip on a Church of England cassock.

Born in Southampton in 1875, Davidson was groomed for a career in the church by his clergyman father. But as a pupil at Whitgift

School, Croydon, south London, he discovered what he considered to be a latent talent for acting. At nineteen he spurned his father's hopes and began work as a stand-up comic, albeit with a scrupulously clean act. Later he went on to win rave reviews for his performance in the title role of a touring production of *Charley's Aunt*.

Yet even as he took the applause of his audience, Davidson's thoughts were very often with the work of the Church. He took to visiting vicars in whichever town his touring company happened to find itself, to ask if they knew any old folk who would like to hear the Bible read out loud. He acquired his interest in helping fallen women after persuading a suicidal teenager not to jump in the Thames. The girl was given some money to return to her home and Davidson went on his way wondering if his true gift wasn't, after all, to do God's work.

By his 22nd birthday he had made up his mind to join the Church. He studied holy orders at Oxford's Exeter College and, though he took five years to pass the three-year degree course, emerged to a curacy at Holy Trinity Church, Windsor. Eight years later he was moved to St-Martin-In-The-Fields, in London, but within twelve months he was on his way to Norfolk to take up the lucrative living of Stiffkey with its £800 salary.

This was more than eight times what his father had first earned and Harold wasted no time setting up a comfortable home. His Irish-born wife, an actress he had met at Oxford, bore him four children. But gossips suggested she didn't really enjoy the role of vicar's wife and the marriage gradually became rocky. By 1913 Davidson was spending most of his working week in London, returning home only to conduct Sunday services, for which he was habitually late.

The reverend's work with poverty-stricken boys in London's East End won him much acclaim, including the congratulations of Queen Mary herself. But in his private life Davidson's odd sexual urges were already beginning to emerge. As chaplain to the Actors' Church Union, he took to lurking in female dressing rooms while actresses stripped for quick costume changes. After several women complained he was banned from a number of theatres.

During World War I Davidson served as a Royal Navy chaplain. He appears to have been best remembered for arranging his church parades at times calculated to inconvenience his superiors. He was also the subject of an embarrassing incident in Cairo when he was arrested during a police raid on a brothel. Davidson insisted he was merely trying to trace a prostitute who was passing venereal diseases among the ratings.

After the war he returned home to discover his wife was pregnant with the child of one of his friends, a colonel he had allowed to live in the vicarage. The marriage was long past saving and Davidson returned to his old habit of spending weekdays in London.

More specifically, his nights were spent in the company of prostitutes – he picked up about 200 a year – and naive young girls. His approach was almost always the same. The woman concerned would be told she looked like a well-known film star and then invited to join him for tea. He got few refusals. Most of the girls saw him as a harmless, quirky old man who just might provide them with some useful contacts in show business.

As the years went by, more and more of Davidson's protégés were invited back to stay at the Stiffkey vicarage. Predictably, his wife Molly was extremely displeased. The family had hit hard times because of Davidson's disastrous business investment in Australian mining and she did not see why they should have to support all these 'lame cats'.

In retrospect, it is amazing that Davidson managed to maintain his job as a country rector for so long. He was eventually trapped by an outraged local magistrate, Major Philip Hammond. Villagers were now gossiping about

'Davidson's girls' and there were regular sightings of them grappling with local youths in a ditch or haystack. Hammond had had enough. He called in the Lord Bishop of Norwich and made a complaint under the Clergy Discipline Act, legislation which allowed wayward vicars suspected of immoral acts to be hauled before a consistory court.

The Bishop at first believed Davidson's work with prostitutes was totally legitimate. But, to play safe, he employed a private detective to check out the reverend's personal life. He could hardly believe the results. The investigation dossier made clear he had to act immediately to preserve the good name of the Church.

Davidson's trial began on 29 March 1932 at Church House in London. The judge, chancellor of the diocese of Norwich, F. Keppel North, presided over weeks of evidence in which a string of nubile young women told how the rector had pestered them under the pretence of caring about their futures. However, the prosecution could produce only one, Barbara Harris, who would accuse him of actually molesting her.

Throughout the hearing, Davidson himself was a poor witness. Just as his defence counsel, Richard Levy, would score a point in his favour, Davidson would undo the good work by appearing contradictory or fatuous. At one point he even denied knowing the meaning of the word 'buttock', a claim which visibly irritated the judge.

His cause was lost when he denied that photographs existed of him with the naked fifteen-year-old daughter of an actress, Mae Douglas. The girl, Estelle Douglas, had wanted to do some modelling work and Davidson had arranged the photographic shoot.

Like lightning, prosecutor Roland Oliver produced a picture showing the girl, her bare bottom towards the camera, posing with a shawl draped around her neck. Davidson's hand was on her right shoulder. Looking flustered and shaken, Davidson hit back by saying the picture was a fake 'touched up' in the darkroom. Then he tried to argue that the shawl had slipped out of his hand "accidentally without my knowledge." Finally he came up with the ludicrous excuse that Estelle been wearing a bathing costume under the shawl a few minutes before the photo was shot. He had not noticed that she had taken it off.

On 8 July 1932 Davidson was found guilty on five counts of immoral conduct and ordered to pay costs. A little over three months later, on 21 October, the Bishop of Norwich announced the rector's defrocking. Davidson, he said, was 'entirely removed, deposed and degraded' from his offices as priest and deacon.

Desperate for cash, Davidson returned to showbusiness – though only just. He earned a living by displaying himself in a barrel on the promenade at Blackpool and would proclaim his innocence to any gawking tripper who happened to pass by.

"The former Rector of Stiffkey," he would bawl, "has been placed in his present position by the authorities of the Church of England who failed in their Christian duty towards him. The lower he sinks, the greater their crime."

It was an awful way to earn a living and it got worse. Davidson varied his act by fasting in a glass box, appearing frozen in a custom-built refrigerator and being roasted alive in a see-through oven while being stabbed with a pitchfork held by a dummy demon.

Eventually Blackpool tired of him and in 1937 he found himself moving to a similar sideshow serving the holidaymakers of Skegness. He played the part of Daniel in the lion's den; no considerable act of courage considering that he was terrified of animals.

But Davidson's days as a novelty act were numbered. On the evening of 28 July, fortified by strong drink, he entered the lions' cage and began poking them with a stick. One of the beasts, Freddy, attacked him and dragged him round the cage by the neck. The audience thought it was all part of the act, until they saw blood oozing from his wounds. Davidson was eventually rescued by the lion tamer's assistant and a member of the public. They were too late to save him. Two days later he died in hospital.

So ended the life of one of England's most bizarre clergymen. The arguments over whether he was a pervert or not have never been settled, nor is there ever likely to be conclusive proof. Yet perhaps the most likely explanation was put forward by the author Tom Cullen in his book *The Prostitute's Padre* (1975). Cullen quotes the rector's long-standing friend J. Rowland Sales, who was convinced Davidson lived out a part-fact-part-fantasy existence as three distinct personas.

One was the kindly clergyman Uncle Harold, another was 'Little Jimmy' who mischievously spent all his spare time getting Uncle Harold into trouble, and the third was 'The Bunco Kid', an unashamed confidence trickster. Davidson, it was argued, spent the later years of his life in a kind of purgatory – torn between all three of his complex identities.

FATTY ARBUCKLE

The party at San Francisco's St Francis Hotel was into its third day and still the guests kept coming. Their host, film comedian Fatty Arbuckle, lapped up the atmosphere, dashing around the suite to ensure everyone had as much food and drink as they wanted. He was enjoying himself. The bash was to celebrate his signing of a $3 million contract and he wasn't about to let such a happy event pass quietly.

That year, 1921, Arbuckle was at the pinnacle of his movie career. Film classics such as *The Sanitarium*, *Fatty's Day Off*, *A Quiet Little Wedding* and *The Masquerader* had catapulted him onto Hollywood's centre stage. By 1916 he was not only starring in films but writing and directing them as well. He went on to set up the production company which gave a good-looking, young hopeful called Buster Keaton his big break in show business.

It wasn't a bad career progression for a guy who started his working life as a plumber's mate. Born Roscoe Conklin Arbuckle in Smith Center, Kansas, on 24 March 1887, Fatty's first experience of acting came on the stages of vaudeville and in small town carnivals. Soon after his 21st birthday he was signed by the Selig

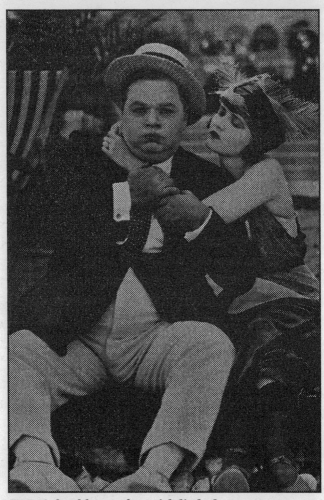

Fatty Arbuckle ... a showgirl died after a party romp in a hotel room.

Polyscope Company as a film extra but within a few months he was angling for bigger parts. In 1910 he got a leading role in *The Sanitarium*, the movie which launched him into the big time. From then on there was no holding him.

Arbuckle was hardly the classical shape for a film legend but his physical attributes got him noticed. Although he had a huge frame of 320 lb he was surprisingly nimble on his feet; a combination which made him naturally funny. His angelic expressions and schoolboy features also marked him down as different, a useful asset even in the early days of the movie business.

With his kind of influence, Arbuckle could have expected to make full use of the casting couch. Yet surprisingly he seems to have rarely made a pass at the bright young things he worked with. Several of them described him as 'brotherly' and 'protective' in his attitude towards them. He certainly had nothing like the romeo reputation that tagged Charlie Chaplin.

Prior to the swinging Twenties there was only one occasion on which Arbuckle found himself almost sucked into scandal.

In 1917 he attended a party in Boston, thrown in his honour by the head of Artcraft production Jesse Lasky. A dozen good-time girls had been provided and at one point several of them jumped onto a table with Fatty to assist him with getting his clothes off.

Unfortunately for the star a nearby resident, curious at the noise, had peeked through a window and witnessed the whole debauched scene. The police were called and threatened to make arrests but rumour has it that Lasky and two associates paid the district attorney and mayor $10,000 to hush things up. Whatever the truth, Arbuckle escaped scot free.

It was to be a very different story at the St Francis Hotel.

That Monday, 5 September 1921, Arbuckle had been keeping an eye out for one guest in particular, a starlet called Virginia Rappe. He had been trying to seduce her for five years, almost from the moment her cherubic face first came to prominence on the cover of the sheet music of *Let Me Call You Sweetheart*. The way she exuded innocence, and her experience as a model in Chicago, had quickly helped her carve out a niche in Hollywood.

In fact Virginia was highly sexed. During her employment with Mack Sennett's film company she slept around so much that production was disrupted and half the staff were obliged to get treatment for crabs.

Sennett was predictably furious and responded by temporarily shutting down his studio and fumigating it.

If Arbuckle knew about this incident it didn't seem to bother him. He'd specifically asked his friend Bambina Maude Delmont to invite Virginia along. Both women were staying at the nearby Palace Hotel with Virginia's agent.

Neither was Fatty deterred by his lack of success in wooing her. Perhaps he hadn't heard her description of him as 'unattractive', or her alleged aside to friends asserting: "I'd sooner go to bed with a jungle ape than have that fat octopus groping at me."

Maybe Fatty thought that the sheer clout he carried in Hollywood would be sufficient to talk her into his bed.

When Virginia arrived Arbuckle was still in his pyjamas, slippers and bathrobe – a style of dress almost de rigeur among the party's long-stayers. They did not meet immediately and it wasn't until she had been handed her third gin and orange, and was complaining to other guests that the bathroom seemed constantly occupied, that Arbuckle whirled into view.

He grabbed her by the arm and with a conspiratorial wink to some friends shepherded her towards the nearest bedroom. Several guests heard him say: "This is what I have been waiting for."

About five minutes later the hubbub of noise in the main suite was abruptly silenced by piercing screams from one of the bedrooms. Maude Delmont grabbed the door and, finding it locked, began shouting: "Virginia, what's happening?"'The screaming persisted and in desperation Maude called the hotel manager's office. The duty manager Mr H.J.Boyle was urgently dispatched to attend to the fracas in room 1219.

Hardly had he got to the door than it burst open and out stepped an amused-looking Arbuckle. He grinned, performed a tap dance on the carpet and tilted Virginia's hat to a drunken angle on his head. Behind him in the room Virginia's groaning was still audible and the sound seemed to irritate Fatty.

"Get her dressed and take her back to the Palace," he snapped at Maude. When Virgina began screaming again he turned his venom on her warning: "Shut up, or I'll throw you out of the window."

Virginia took no notice. As Boyle and Maude dashed to her side she murmured: "I'm dying, I'm dying. He hurt me."

She was almost naked and it was difficult to get her dressed. Her badly ripped blouse had been torn off her body.

Arbuckle seemed oblivious to the drama. His dismissive attitude left guests in no doubt that he suspected Virginia of 'putting it on' – maybe even to cajole him into giving her a good part. "Shut up," he bellowed at her. "You always were a lousy actress."

Three days later Virginia died of peritonitis. An autopsy showed her full bladder had burst, an injury which may have occurred when Arbuckle threw his bulk on top of her.

The papers immediately began talking of him as a sex fiend who threw orgies as a matter of course and was guilty of rape. There were untrue rumours that his manhood was so large that it had penetrated Virginia's bladder in the act of intercourse. Arbuckle's friend Al Seminacher fuelled even wilder gossip by suggesting the star had pushed a large ice cube up her vagina and sexually assaulted her with a champagne bottle.

An inquest decided Arbuckle was 'criminally responsible' for her death and he was later charged with manslaughter.

In the eyes of his public he was already guilty. Church leaders demanded a ban on his films, women's groups expressed outrage and in Wyoming a group of cowboys peppered a movie screen with bullets because it was showing a Fatty 'short'.

At his trial in November 1921, Arbuckle angrily refuted the charge against him. His lawyers claimed Virginia Rappe was little more than a common prostitute and they got most of the jury on his side. But the majority ten-to-two vote in Fatty's favour was insufficient to get an acquittal.

A new trial was held in which jurors concluded just the opposite, voting ten to two that he was guilty.

Eventually, he was cleared at the third attempt. The jury foreman told the judge: "Acquittal is not enough. We feel a grave injustice has been done to him and there is not the slightest proof to connect him in any way with the commission of a crime."

Arbuckle emerged from court to tell the reporters who had crucified him: "My innocence of the hideous charge preferred against me has been proved."

It was a statement delivered more out of bravado than any real conviction. Arbuckle's lawyers must have told him it that it is almost impossible to 'prove' a negative: that is, that a particular event never happened. The mud had stuck and Fatty's public could no longer laugh at him. His career was in tatters.

The $3 million contract was torn up and for the next ten years he lived the life of a second-string actor, touring small theatres in the sticks for pay amounting to peanuts. In one interview for *Photoplay* magazine he begged: "Just let me work. I think I can entertain and gladden the people that see me."

Finally in June 1933 he seized his comeback chance. Warner Brothers signed him to make a series of comedy shorts and, with some trepidation, threw a celebration party in his honour at a hotel in New York.

The bash ended with another tragic death. They found Fatty Arbuckle in his room, the victim of a massive coronary. He was just 46 years old.

CHARLIE CHAPLIN

To millions of his fans, Charlie Chaplin was simply the greatest silent movie actor of a generation. His blend of clowning and pathos marked him out as comic genius and his dark, soulful eyes had women swooning wherever his films were shown. Those who saw classics such as *The Rink*, *Easy Street*, *The Cure*, *The Immigrant* and *The Kid* believed in the hapless little tramp and his crazy adventures. In the early days of his career, the idea of Chaplin embroiled in a sex scandal was akin to the prospect of Fatty Arbuckle selling slimming aids.

Yet between the wars, Chaplin's private life was increasingly dissected and devoured by a scandal-hungry press. The tramp, it seemed, had penchants for threesomes, fellatio, and performing intercourse in front of spectators. Above all, he liked sex with schoolgirls.

There was more. Before he hit the big time Chaplin would venture out with showbusiness friends from vaudeville to frequent brothels. At twenty, he once baulked at paying the asking price to an experienced Parisian prostitute and ran off before they got to her apartment. Yet prostitutes were only an idle distraction in his highly active sex life. He pursued and seduced

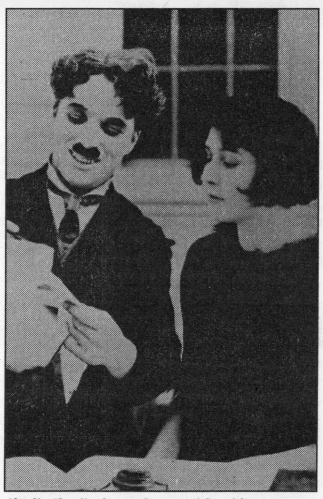

Charlie Chaplin, lover of young girls, with co-star
Paulette Goddard.

many notable women including Winston Churchill's cousin Clare Sheridan, Ziegfeld girl Peggy Hopkins Joyce (with whom he delighted in swimming nude off the isle of Catalina), and actresses Mabel Normand, Edna Purviance, Pola Negri and Marion Davies.

Rumour had it that he was also a keen voyeur. He was said to have set up a telescope at his house to provide close up views of his neighbour John Barrymore's bedroom. It was all part of a complex sexual philosophy. "No art can be learned at once," he would tell his friends. "And lovemaking is a sublime art that needs practice if it is to be true and significant."

Chaplin was 29 when he took his first bride to the altar in 1918. But that marriage to 16-year-old film extra Mildred Harris was doomed, and the pair divorced two years later.

The next Mrs Chaplin was another 16-year-old, Lolita MacMurray. She later changed her name by deed poll to Lita Grey, hoping it would help secure her a career in films. Though that union, sealed in 1924, produced Charlie's sons Charles and Sydney, the marriage again spun into trouble. The bitter divorce case ended with a multi-million dollar settlement against Chaplin.

The resulting publicity was devoured by Hollywood. Lita's divorce papers, filed in 1926, were published and touted on the streets for a quarter of a dollar a copy. They revealed how Charlie had sex with at least five mistresses during the marriage, how he tried to talk her into a bedroom threesome, how he would wave a loaded gun in front of her face, how he wanted them to copulate in front of an audience and how he repeatedly demanded that she perform fellatio on him. Chaplin argued that 'all married people do it'. Lita told him he was a pervert.

In her autobiography, she later described how Chaplin molested her when she was just fifteen during the filming of *The Gold Rush*. "He kissed my mouth and neck and his fingers darted over my alarmed body," she wrote. "His body writhed furiously against mine and suddenly some of my fright gave way to revulsion."

Once, when Lita commented that he could have his pick of any one of a hundred women in two minutes, Charlie replied: "A hundred? No, a thousand. But I want to be naughty with you, not with them."

Chaplin's third marriage, to twenty-year-old starlet Paulette Goddard, has remained shrouded in mystery. Some claim the ceremony took place aboard his yacht *Panacea* in 1934 and that Chaplin ordered his skipper to tear out the log record. Chaplin himself insisted that they wed in 1936. Either way the match quickly went the way of his previous marriages and ended in 1942.

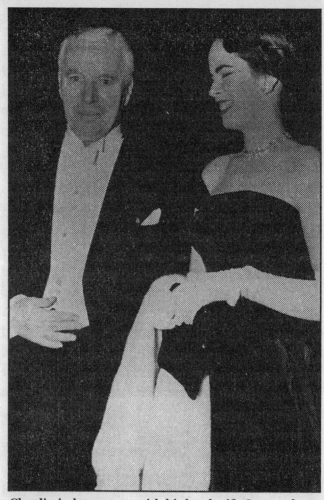

Chaplin in later years with his loyal wife Oona, whom he wed when she was seventeen.

Hardly had Goddard's divorce papers been filed, than the scandal for which Chaplin became notorious broke in the press. An ambitious young actress called Joan Barry alleged that he had bedded her at fifteen and that she was carrying his love child. One of Hollywood's biggest names was suddenly facing criminal proceedings. The charge, linked to Federal anti-prostitution laws, was that Chaplin had transported a minor across state lines for immoral purposes.

Barry claimed her fling with the star lasted well into the autumn of 1942. He had promised to make her a leading lady, and paid for her to receive singing and acting lessons. Even after the relationship turned sour they had indulged their lust in the most bizarre ways. Barry claimed that during Christmas 1942 she forced her way into Chaplin's Californian home pointing a gun at him. The incident aroused the couple's sense of eroticism and they copulated in the bedroom. But he pressed charges and she was given a 30-day jail sentence for unlawfully entering his house.

On her release, Barry poured out the whole sordid story to Hollywood's most notorious gossip columnist, Hedda Hopper. Hopper had long loathed Chaplin for his rumoured liaisons with minors, his renowned left-wing and Russian sympathies and his dogged refusal to seek full American citizenship. Now she had the ammunition she needed to vilify him in public.

She ran a series of articles suggesting that Chaplin was the father of Joan Barry's unborn child. He responded by putting off a proposed marriage to his fourth wife, the seventeen-year-old Oona O'Neil and embarked on a damage limitation exercise to try and save his reputation. It failed. In June 1943 Barry filed her paternity suit.

Before it could be heard however, Chaplin had to fight the FBI prosecution alleging that he had brought Barry across state boundaries to New York specifically to have intercourse with her. He hired leading lawyer Jerry Giesler, unofficial attorney-to-the-stars, and Giesler turned in his usual masterly performance. He argued that Charlie and Joan had enjoyed a private romance and that it was at no time necessary for him to ferry her around the country for sex. The jury agreed and Chaplin walked free. But now his reputation was permanently tarnished. Public sympathy was running against him.

Joan's child, Carol Ann, was born on 2 October 1943 and she milked every ounce of publicity she could out of the event. When the paternity suit at last came to court in December of the following year, she ensured Carol Ann was with her every day. In the eyes of the jury, this undoubtably promoted her case as a lone mother abandoned by a heartless, wealthy film star. They were also impressed by the firebrand prosecutor who referred to Chaplin in court as 'a runt of a Svengali' and a 'lecherous hound'.

Yet blood tests carried out on Chaplin showed he was not the child's father. His lawyers argued that Joan had indulged in affairs with at least one other man during her relationship with Charlie. Some of her travelling expenses, it was claimed, had been met by the oil tycoon J. Paul Getty. The inference was clear but it was not backed by a shred of proof.

When a mis-trial was announced it seemed Chaplin had escaped. However, in a weird judicial twist, the court decided that he should pay a substantial, undisclosed sum towards the child's maintenance. Public opinion held that this was the very least the star should expect. Continuing rumours about his red-under-the-bed tendencies and hints that he was a tax evader prompted outrage among patriotic Americans. They boycotted his 1947 film *Monsieur Verdoux* in their thousands and though it was hailed an artistic triumph by the critics it was a financial flop. Chaplin began to see that he would not easily be forgiven for his indiscretions.

In 1952 he left the US with Oona and his children for a holiday in Switzerland. He probably knew that his re-entry to America would be challenged by the government and he made no attempt to return. Instead he declared himself a 'citizen of the world' and made a permanent residence in Switzerland.

He returned to the US only once – in 1972 – to receive an honorary Oscar in recognition of his contribution to the movie business. He got another academy award the following year for his score of *Limelight*, released in 1952.

Chaplin died in 1977, now fully rehabilitated by Hollywood. Of Joan Barry, little was heard after she was committed to a Californian mental hospital in 1953. Her daughter, Carol Ann Chaplin, has consistently maintained a low public profile.

KING EDWARD VIII AND WALLIS SIMPSON

The question directed across the floor of the House of Commons by socialist MP Ellen Wilkinson was carefully crafted. To most of the British public it seemed he was concerning himself only with an unusual aspect of censorship affecting imported American magazines. But to a privileged few, dipping into the cauldron of gossip stirred by Westminster and the newspapers, Wilkinson's phraseology meant much more. He had just attempted a peek behind the cloak of secrecy surrounding the greatest royal scandal of the twentieth century: the love affair of King Edward VIII and American divorcee Wallis Simpson.

Wilkinson's question that afternoon, 17 November 1936, was directed at the President of the Board of Trade, Sir Walter Runciman. "Can the Right Honourable Gentleman say why," he asked, "in the case of two American magazines of the highest repute imported into this country in the last few weeks, two and sometimes three pages have been torn out; and what is this thing the British public are not allowed to know?" Runciman responded with the classic political get-out: "My department has nothing to do with that."

In fact, for months newspapers and magazines outside the UK had been reporting the scurrilous gossip surrounding the new king and Mrs Simpson. How they had met in 1930 at a cocktail party thrown by the American-born Lady Thelma Furness in London's Grosvenor Square. How Edward, then Prince of Wales, had invited her to his retreat at Fort Belvedere in Windsor Great Park. And how by 1935 Wallis and Edward had been seen holidaying together on a Mediterranean cruise, tasting the mountain air in Switzerland, Austria and Hungary, and soaking up sunshine in the south of France.

On every occasion care was taken to extend the king's hospitality to her husband Ernest, a wealthy international shipbroker of Anglo-American stock. But the foreign journalists sniffing hard around the story were familiar with the posturings of the rich and famous. Every invitation from Buckingham Palace received a polite refusal from Ernest, usually on the grounds that he was too busy at work. With each refusal came Wallis's acceptance. And with each of her visits the scandal grew.

Yet it wasn't until 20 January 1936 that the crisis began to break. On that date King George V died and his son and heir, the 41-year-old

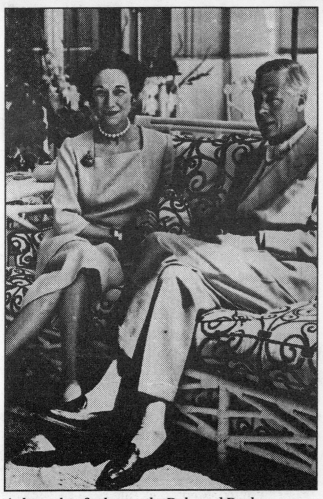

A throne lost for love ... the Duke and Duchess of Windsor.

Edward Albert Christian George Andrew Patrick David Windsor (plain 'David' in royal circles) took the throne. Almost immediately he started formulating a plan to have the lady he loved crowned queen at his side.

So who was this woman who so captivated a king? And what was the bewitching power she appeared to hold over him.

There was indeed much more to 39-year-old Wallis, the woman from Blue Ridge Summit, Pennsylvania, than met the eye. And a great deal of her life story was known to British Intelligence.

The men of MI6 were particularly interested in the time she had spent in China and Hong Kong with her first husband, US naval pilot Lieutenant Earl Winfield Spencer. During his posting there in the mid-twenties the couple had frequented the Far East's legendary brothels, the 'Singing Houses' as they were known. Wallis had been transfixed by the orgies and the lovemaking techniques used by teenage prostitutes. She joined in some of their sex games, anxious to learn 'fang yung', a sexual foreplay that involved the massage of every part of a man's body. It was rumoured to produce an explosive sexual performance.

MI6 included it all in the 'China Report' a complete dossier of Wallis's sexual indiscretions which had been presented to Edward's father and

Prime Minister Stanley Baldwin. A quick scan through its pages made one thing certain in their minds. This woman could never be Queen of England.

Wallis was said to wield a bizarre personal and sexual dominance over Edward. Allegedly she indulged in regular sadistic practices, whipping him across the buttocks using a short riding crop. Edward was apparently a willing participant and his staff would, on occasions, find his underpants streaked with blood.

As the inevitable royal marriage conflict with Parliament approached, the king was clear in his own mind what needed to be done. He was set on having Wallis crowned with him on the date set for his Coronation, 12 May 1937. However, for this timescale to be accomplished Wallis needed to ensure an uncontested 'quickie' divorce. She could then be granted a 'decree absolute' by the British courts and be free to re-marry within six months.

The king personally managed the divorce proceedings. He agreed to a meeting with Ernest Simpson one evening in February 1936 at which Simpson asked him: "Are you sincere? Do you intend to marry her?" At this the king replied: "Do you really think I would be crowned without Wallis by my side?"

The two men struck a bargain ensuring the

marriage break was clean, and parted on reasonably amicable terms.

Perhaps this turn of events left Edward over-confident. In any case his decision to take Wallis with him on a summer cruise of the Mediterranean was seen as both unwise and reckless by politicians and Palace aides alike. The trip triggered worldwide publicity as the couple were photographed and courted at every port of call.

Back home Fleet Street was losing patience. Editors had agreed to respect the monarch's privacy on holiday but they failed to see why their readers should be denied information freely available to the rest of the world. No newspaper openly referred to Wallis's presence aboard the royal yacht, though *The Times* fulminated that sovereigns 'should be invested with a certain detachment and dignity'.

On October 12 the most powerful newspaper baron in the country, Canadian Lord Beaver-brook, discovered that the Simpsons' divorce petition was to be heard at Ipswich.

He warned Wallis' solicitor, Theodore Goddard, that he intended to publish a report, but was dissuaded after the king himself asked for Beaverbrook's help in limiting publicity. Edward argued that his 'friend' was 'ill, unhappy and distressed by the thought of notoriety'.

Beaverbrook succeeded in securing an unprecedented pact from other newspaper proprietors and the divorce went duly unreported. Wallis was granted a decree nisi on the grounds of her husband's adultery with an unnamed woman, who was actually a professional divorce co-respondent called Buttercup Kennedy. Yet just as the king might have thought a crucial hurdle had been safely negotiated, the crisis that would end in his abdication was ignited.

On 13 November the king opened a peremptory letter from his Private Secretary, Major Alexander Hardinge. Hardinge warned that the Cabinet was about to debate the royal love affair, and that unless its advice was taken the government was prepared to fight an election on the Edward and Mrs Simpson issue.

The letter continued: "If Your Majesty will permit me to say so, there is only one step which holds out any prospect of avoiding this dangerous situation, and that is for Mrs Simpson to go abroad without further delay and I would beg Your Majesty to give this proposal your earnest consideration before the situation becomes irretrievable."

The king rejected the suggestion. He prepared to face Prime Minister Baldwin with the argument that he and Wallis should have a morganatic marriage; that is, one in which neither she nor their children would have any claim to a royal title and would be barred from entering the line of succession.

Baldwin realised this would be unacceptable to both Parliament and the governments of the Dominions, who, by law, had a right to veto any proposed alterations to the Succession. When he canvassed the individual governments by telegram he received the emphatic rejection he had expected.

At the end of November the scandal exploded, shocking a bemused British public. The Cabinet rejected the morganatic marriage solution and the story of the royal love affair was recounted in a tidal wave of newsprint. Editors pegged their stories on a speech by the Bishop of Bradford, Dr Alfred Blunt, in which he suggested the king needed to show 'more positive awareness' of his duty to God and country.

Now Baldwin confronted Edward with three choices. Either he forget the marriage completely, marry against the advice of his ministers and spark a constitutional crisis or abdicate and marry.

Baldwin insists he was against abdication but, he recalled later, the king's response was: "You want me to go don't you? And before I go, I think it is right for her sake and mine that I should speak."

Baldwin coldly replied: "What I want, sir, is what you told me you wanted: to go with dignity, not dividing the country, and making things as smooth as possible for your successor. You will be telling millions throughout the world, among them a vast number of women, that you are determined to marry one who has a husband living. You may, by speaking, divide opinion; but you will certainly harden it."

Later the king left Buckingham Palace for the last time as monarch and headed for Fort Belvedere. If he had been in any doubt of Baldwin's advice, the reaction of Parliament to a speech by the Premier on 5 December must have settled it. Baldwin told the House that a morganatic marriage did not have any basis in English law.

"The lady whom he (the king) marries necessarily becomes queen," he said. "The only way in which this result could be avoided would be by legislation dealing with a particular case. His Majesty's Government are not prepared to introduce such legislation." At those words almost the entire House erupted in loud cheering.

The following day Edward informed Baldwin of his decision to abdicate and despite desperate attempts to persuade him to think again, he would not be moved.

On 10 December he signed the Instrument of Abdication renouncing all claims on the British throne. The following day he spoke during a BBC broadcast which, for seventy historic seconds, brought every corner of the English-speaking world to a hushed standstill.

In a faltering voice, he said: "You all know the reasons which have impelled me to renounce the Throne. But I want you to understand that in making up my mind I did not forget the country or the empire which as Prince of Wales, and lately as king, I have for 25 years tried to serve. But you must believe me when I tell you that I have found it impossible to carry the heavy burden of responsibility and to discharge my duties as king as I would wish to do, without the help and support of the woman I love."

On the night of 11 December Edward sailed into exile aboard a British destroyer. He and Wallis married quietly at the Chateau de Cande, near Tours, in June 1937. There were no members of the Royal Family present and the service was conducted by an unknown, unidentified volunteer priest from Darlington.

Edward's 'damnable wedding present', as he called it, from the British government was the announcement that his future title would be His Royal Highness the Duke of Windsor. Wallis however was to be denied use of the

HRH initials she wanted so badly. She was to be known simply as the Duchess of Windsor, confirming her status as a commoner in the eyes of the Establishment.

The Duke died of throat cancer in 1972. His wife survived him for fourteen lonely years, regarded as an outcast by the Royal Family and a curiosity by the gossip columnists. She was buried beside the man she loved at Frogmore, Windsor, in April 1986.

LADY DIANA DELVES BROUGHTON (THE HAPPY VALLEY MURDER)

The body of Josslyn Victor Hay, 22nd Earl of Erroll, Baron Kilmarnock, Hereditary High Constable of Scotland, was found slumped under the dashboard of his car on the Nairobi-Ngong road in Kenya. He had been shot. The discovery was made at three o'clock in the morning by the native driver of a milk truck. Police were called and the local pathologist, who happened to be driving past the spot on his way to work, hauled the corpse from the car at 8am. He immediately recognised the dead man as one of the leading lights of the expatriate community in Kenya – and one of the country's biggest murder hunts was set in motion.

The date was 24 January 1941. Yet to this day no one has ever been convicted of the murder.

The killing of Josslyn Hay occurred in Kenya's White Highlands – nicknamed Happy Valley because of its natural beauty and because of the hedonistic pleasures enjoyed by its wealthy inhabitants. More than 3,000 miles away from war-torn England, the Happy Valley set could have been on a different planet. Certainly they formed a society from a different age. Flamboyant, drink-swilling, sexually licentious cocaine snorters, they were described by a contemporary writer as 'having libidos matched only by their unquenchable thirst for fine champagne, cognac and wines'. Foremost among them was old Etonian Josslyn Hay, known as the 'Passionate Peer' because of his amorous adventures.

Hay, at 39 years of age, was a suave, handsome philanderer whose favourite catchphrase was 'to hell with husbands'. That was his philosophy as he held court at the gracious Muthaiga Country Club, scene of bawdy parties, nights of drunken revelry and drug-taking. Among the Happy Valley set his reputation was as an accomplished seducer.

Hay worked as a military secretary at a time when Kenya was an all-important strategic mustering point for British forces planning the assault on Ethiopia, then under the control of Mussolini's fascists.

Despite having been expelled from Eton for bad behaviour and later being cited in a divorce case in which the judge called him 'a very bad blackguard', Josslyn Hay seemed to have landed on his feet as an administrator of one of the jewels in Britain's colonial crown. His days were spent writing languid memos to his Whitehall superiors. The nights he reserved for womanising.

Hay cut a dashing figure at the Muthaiga Club. In his Saville Row evening suit, the smoke trailing lazily from his Turkish cigarettes, he was the ultimate lounge lizard.

For women whose husbands were incredibly wealthy, there was little to do but find diversion with interesting and interested men. Hay was such a man. And just such a woman was Lady Diana Delves Broughton, a beauty with an English rose complexion who, at 26, was 30 years younger than her husband. He was property magnate and racing fanatic Sir Henry Delves Broughton, known to his expatriate pals simply as 'Jock'.

Josslyn and Diana met on 30 November 1940 at the Muthaiga Club. He later told friends:

"Never can I remember a woman having such an immediate impact on me. I saw her eyes boring into me and I knew then that I must have her. I walked over to her while Jock was at the bar and said to her, 'Well, who is going to tell Jock – you or I?'"

Diana was entranced by the master seducer. It was not long before they were seen dining out together, attending dances at the colonial clubs, taking tea on the terraces and enjoying risqué weekends at the homes of friends who could be trusted. Both became willing participants in the passion which would eventually lead to murder.

Sir Henry, who had married Diana only weeks before emigrating to Kenya, had struck an extraordinary pact with her, promising not to stand in her way if she fell in love with a younger man – and to pay several thousand pounds annually to her for some years after their divorce. But he could hardly have expected that their marriage would founder within so short a time.

Gossip was rife about the affair between his wife and Hay. A note was even left at the club asking him what he planned to do about the eternal triangle. Another anonymous note was delivered on the day Diana left for an 'all girls' swimming party outing to Nyeri. The note informed Sir Henry that there were no girls on the outing – only Josslyn Hay. Despite his stiff-upper-lip stoicism (he was also an old Etonian), Sir Henry resolved to act.

On 18 January, his wife told Delves Broughton that she was madly in love with Joss and that she wanted to leave him. Recalling his own marriage pledge and its promise of her freedom, Sir Henry offered to take her on a three-month trip to Ceylon. Bizarrely, he offered that if she would reconsider her feelings on the journey, she could bring Hay along.

Diana rejected her husband's offer. Two days later she walked out on him, saying that she was going to live with Hay. She took with her a £5,000 string of pearls, which her husband had ordered from Asprey's, the London jewellers, as an inducement for her to stay.

Three days later, Delves Broughton rang the police and reported a burglary, saying that two revolvers, some money and a cigarette case had been stolen. That same day he saw his lawyers about a divorce and later wrote to a friend:

"They say they are in love with each other and mean to get married. It is a hopeless position and I'm going to cut my losses. I think I'll go to Ceylon. There's nothing for me to live in Kenya for."

The following day he received another anonymous note, this one reading:

"There's no fool like an old fool. What are you going to do about it?"

As Diana moved into Hay's colonial mansion, where they made love on silk sheets monogrammed with his family crest, some of Jock's friends, fearing for his emotional state, began to rally round and comfort him. One of these, a Mrs Carberry, invited him to tea on 23 January. Unfortunately, Diana and Hay turned up unexpectedly – part of the latter's wicked manoeuvrings aimed at making his mistress's husband suffer.

However, Jock's demeanour disappointed Hay at the tea. It was a set piece of English politeness, of stiff upper lips and no mention of broken hearts and betrayed passions. Afterwards, Lord Errol told a friend:

"Jock could not have been nicer. He has agreed to go away. As a matter of fact he has been so nice it smells bad."

That night there was more largesse on the part of Delves Broughton. At a dinner party at the club, where by now everyone knew of the steamy affair, the cuckolded husband raised his glass in a toast and declared:

"I wish them every happiness. May their union be blessed with an heir. To Diana and Joss."

At about 2am, slightly the worse for wear, having imbibed huge quantities of champagne, Delves Broughton returned to his house. Hay promised to deliver Diana safely home, and at 2.15 am he dropped her off in his Buick.

At 3am the body of Josslyn Hay was found slumped under the dashboard of the car, which had left the road and plunged into a ditch only three miles from Delves Broughton's home. It was no accident: he had been shot through the head at point-blank range with a .32 revolver.

On 25 January, Josslyn Hay was buried – and

it was only then that the police announced that he had been murdered. They said that someone had either flagged the car down, had been sitting beside the driver, or had fired a shot through the open window from the running board.

Diana, who had to be sedated because of her grief at her lover's death, now accused her husband of cold-bloodedly killing him out of jealousy. But for some reason she relented, and by the time police formally charged him with the murder she had flown to Johannesburg to hire him top criminal lawyer Harry Morris. It was a worthwhile investment.

Morris called experts to prove that the three bullets fired at Josslyn Hay could not have come from any gun owned by Delves Broughton. The accused performed masterfully in the dock. Of the love trysts that continued under his own roof, he said resignedly:

"She could ask who she liked. I should not have tried to stop her in any event. I see no point in it. We met every day at the club and I cannot see it makes any difference if a man comes to stay the night."

"In my experience of life, if you try to stop a woman doing anything, she wants to do it all the more. With a young wife the only thing to do is keep her amused."

On 1 July 1941 Delves Broughton was found

not guilty. He took Diana on their planned trip to Ceylon before returning to England, ailing and partially paralysed. He committed suicide in Liverpool on 5 December 1942, leaving notes which said he had found the strain of the trial and accompanying publicity too much to bear.

Diana stayed on in Kenya until the end of her life in 1987. The file on the murder has never been closed because the killer has never been caught.

ERROL FLYNN

The sexual exploits of Australian hellraiser Errol Flynn began at an early age. He was seventeen when he was kicked out of school after being caught with the daughter of a laundress.

After turning to acting, he was brought to Hollywood where he described himself as a walking phallic symbol. He defied the Hollywood morality of the time and was infamous for his boozing, fighting and womanising. When he attained fame and fortune, he bought a yacht named *Cirrhosis By The Sea* and moved to a house in the Hollywood Hills which he equipped with an orgy room.

When it was put up for sale in 1978 it was discovered that the bedrooms were fitted with two-way mirrors and microphones. He and guests at his bawdy parties would would watch as other couples paired off for sex romps.

"The orgies that went on there would make Hollywood today look like a Sunday school," a real estate agent said at the time.

"He would change women as quickly as his valet could change the sheets," said his second wife Nora Eddington.

On the day of his marriage in Monaco to his

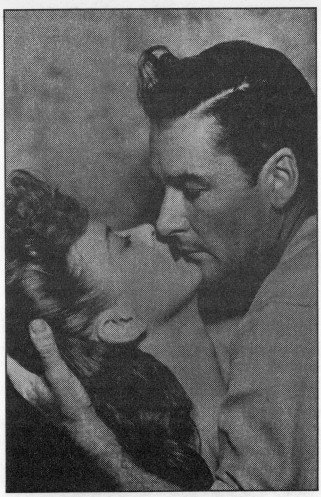

Heart-throb Errol Flynn was an even wilder lover off-screen.

third wife, Patrice Wymore, he was arrested on the steps of the church for the alleged rape of a seventeen-year-old girl. The charge was dropped after the two came face to face in a police station, Flynn later recalling:

"As soon as I saw her hairy legs I knew I was innocent."

Drunk, sober, drugged or partly insane, these were not the legs Flynn would have had next to his.

However, two further, sordid rape cases did shatter Flynn's career. The movie star was 33 when two young girls laid complaints against him with Hollywood police. One said he had ravished her by land, the other girl claimed it was on his yacht.

He went into court in 1943 charged with statutory rape, the Californian legal term for sex with a minor.

The trial was a farce. Nightclub dancer Peggy 'La Rue' Satterlee appeared in court in pigtails and bobbysocks, attempting to persuade the jury that she was under eighteen at the time of the alleged offence. A second girl, seventeen-year-old shop assistant Betty Hansen, caused laughter in the court when she told how Flynn had undressed her apart from her socks, then climbed into bed with only his boots on.

After hearing the evidence against himself,

Flynn said:

"I was attacked as a sex criminal. I knew I could never escape this brand, that I would always be associated in the public mind with an internationally followed rape case."

He was right. Although he won the case and enjoyed a brief period of notoriety, his long-term film career was finished. He did not work at all for a year and the scandal plummeted him into a world of drugs and alcohol. Flynn died of a heart attack in 1959 at the age of 50.

ROCK HUDSON

The world's press was gathered in the street outside the American Hospital in Paris. Inside was one of Hollywood's greatest heart-throbs – a manly love god, envied by men and lusted after by women. His publicity girl came to the hospital door and the newsmen leapt forward to interrogate her. What, they wanted to know, was wrong with Rock Hudson?

Softly, publicist Yanou Collart answered: "Mr Hudson has Acquired Immune Deficiency Syndrome. It was diagnosed over a year ago in the United States."

The media men stood for a moment in shocked silence. Then they raced to telephones to tell the world that the 59-year-old hunk was the first major celebrity to contract AIDS. It was to be a shocking end for one of the silver screen's most dashing hunks.

Rock Hudson's entire life was a fiction managed by Hollywood. Born Roy Fitzgerald, he grew up with an abandoned mother he adored and a stepfather he hated. He was a Navy veteran, truck driver and vacuum cleaner salesman before leaving his home town of Winnetka, Illinois, for the sparkling lights of Hollywood.

There he gravitated to the gay community of Long Beach, where he felt completely at ease. It was there he met talent scout Henry Willson, who renamed his latest discovery Rock Hudson – after the Rock of Gibraltar and the Hudson River. The legend had been born. But the myth of the Adonis, the lady-killer with strapping masculinity, had to be maintained.

It was not easy. Studio chiefs went to amazing lengths to disguise his sexual liaisons. When he fell madly in love with one young man, scandal threatened. Hudson was ordered to drop him, and the star did not live with another man for ten years. Finally, a marriage was arranged. The studio decided that the 'lucky' bride should be his agent's secretary, Phyllis Gates.

The ceremony took place on 9 November 1955 and went ahead even though neither Rock nor the studio had bothered to tell the blushing bride that it was a set-up – or even that her husband was gay. Thereafter, Phyllis Gates was utterly frustrated and perplexed at Hudson's lack of sexual interest in her. She even consulted a psychiatrist who suggested she wear frilly underwear to seduce her husband! An even sadder side to their relationship emerged after his death, when she revealed that he beat her, probably out of his own frustration at his entrapment in a sham marriage.

None of this surfaced at the time, of course, and Rock's career continued to soar above most other stars. By 1960, when he made the memorable comedy *Pillow Talk* with his good friend Doris Day, Hudson was one of the world's biggest box office attractions. As his career hit the stratosphere, Rock began to think more and more about sex and less and less about acting. He said that he thought about sex constantly, even when rehearsing his lines or driving to the studio.

Thoughts became deeds. His sexual energy was rumoured to be so enormous that he could have sex sessions with several people, several times a day. When he entertained at his Beverly Hills estate, known as The Castle, he would always have several handsome young men frolicking in the pool to choose from.

In 1973 publicist Tom Clark moved into The Castle. Clark was a far cry from the pretty-faced men he usually dated. But he enjoyed the same hobbies of football, cooking and travelling that Rock did, and became the great love of the star's life. As a bonus, for the first time Hudson could actually take a man with him everywhere he wished – for Tom Clark had become the actor's manager.

The two lovers hosted many lavish parties at the estate, including one for Rock's 50th birthday in 1975. On this occasion, the star walked down the staircase clad only in a nappy, while the band played *You Must Have Been a Beautiful Baby*. "It was," Rock recalled, "the prettiest party we ever had."

As the 1980s dawned, however, Rock's love of parties – and his growing love of the bottle – were taking their toll on his health and his appearance.

In 1982 Hudson tired of his long-time lover, Tom Clark. Within a year, a new man replaced him in Rock's affections: 29-year-old Marc Christian, whom he had met at a charity event in Los Angeles. The pair met in out-of-the-way restaurants, and after a year of their first date Marc moved into The Castle and into Rock's bed. The love-struck star gave Marc a new Cadillac to replace his 26-year-old car. He also gave him the run of his mansion.

Rock Hudson's once-unstoppable movie career faltered, as his looks began to betray his hectic lifestyle, though he managed to become a regular in the television saga *Dynasty*. By now he had AIDS - and he knew it. But selfishly he wasn't telling anyone, not even Marc Christian.

In July 1985 Rock flew to Paris for treatment. He was so weak that he collapsed in his suite at The Ritz and was rushed to the American Hospital. From there, he authorised the statement finally admitting that he was suffering from AIDS. Marc Christian heard the shock announcement on the six o'clock TV news. Until then, he had believed his star lover's denials that he had the disease.

Rock Hudson was flown back to Los Angeles on a chartered jet, from which he was removed by stretcher at dead of night. His wraith-like frame was taken by helicopter to the University of California Medical Center but there was little the specialists could do. Reunited with Marc back at The Castle, he took short walks beside the pool and would gaze out over the city. "He would look at that view and go off into another world," said Christian. "I guess he was wondering how all of this happened."

When he wasn't feeling well enough for his walks, he would sit and watch old movies, especially those staring Bette Davis. Until the last two weeks of his life, during which his condition grew rapidly worse, he received no specific treatment for his illness. There was virtually nothing anyone could do to ease his distressing condition.

His regular companions at this time were his old friend Liz Taylor and his ex-lover Tom Clark, who moved back into The Castle to care for him. At Clark's request, a priest visited the estate, gave Rock communion and took his confession.

On the morning of 2 October 1985 Rock awoke early. A nurse dressed him – with difficulty, because he was receiving nourishment through an intravenous drip. Clark watched over him and realised that his condition was worsening. He undressed him again and put him back to bed. Within half an hour, he was dead.

The scandals surrounding Rock Hudson's demise failed to die with him. Marc Christian, cut out of the star's will, launched a lawsuit against his estate, claiming that his lover, friends and doctors had withheld potentially life-saving information from him. "I moved into Rock Hudson's house and trusted him," Marc told a court. "I want justice." Finally, in June 1991, an appeals court upheld a $5 million award to Marc to compensate for the fear of his developing AIDS, which a judge described as "the ultimate in personal horror".

LORD LAMBTON

For centuries, politicians embroiled in scandal have tried to live by the maxim: 'Do as I say; not as I do.' Only when their seedy deeds become public is there any evidence of contrition, and even then it is often tainted with self-righteous speeches.

Double standards seem to be fine ... as long as you don't get caught.

The case of Lord Lambton is the perfect illustration of how a typical British Establishment figure reacts to scandal. His is a sordid tale of prostitution, deception and manipulation in which none of the main players emerge with a shred of credit.

Lambton first took his seat in the House of Commons in 1951 after his father's influence helped propel him into the safe Conservative seat of Berwick-on-Tweed.

Though only 28 – an infant in Parliamentary terms – he quickly rose through the ranks, obtaining a succession of ministerial posts. Having been told of the Profumo affair, in which the Minister for War, John Profumo, was caught with a call girl, Christine Keeler, Lambton wrote a pompous, holier-than-thou type letter to a newspaper.

It included words that would return to haunt him:

"I warned the Conservative Party but no-one took any notice. One cannot help regretting the whole of this squalid affair. It is the beginning of another unfortunate chapter which may end heaven knows where."

On the death of his father in 1970 Anthony Lambton inherited the title Earl of Durham, an event which forced him to reassess his own political future. Under British constitutional law, he could no longer remain a Member of Parliament and retain his title.

He had two choices: either to become the sixth earl, resign from the Commons and take his ancestral seat in the House of Lords, or to renounce the earldom and carve himself a slice of real power in the Commons.

Lambton chose the latter course. But his years of breeding and sense of aristocratic tradition did not always sit well with his new role as a commoner.

When MPs decided in 1972 to abandon the practice of using titles in the Commons chamber, he rebelled and insisted that he should continue to be called Lord Lambton.

However, Lambton was neither a social snob nor the product of a sheltered upbringing. He became heir to the earldom only after the tragic death of his elder brother, John, in a shooting accident.

That same year, 1940, he was steered into an army career and began officer training at Sandhurst. But the combination of an asthma condition and bad eyesight meant he was invalided out before long .

For the next five years he was employed as a fitter in a Tyneside shipyard alongside many workmates who were tenants on his father's land.

During the war he met and married the nineteen-year-old Belinda Blew-Jones, daughter of a retired army officer.

The marriage was a strong one and the couple immediately set about their family duty of producing an heir.

It proved a difficult task. After fifteen years their brood comprised five daughters and it was not until 1961 that a son, Edward, was born. Lambton celebrated by throwing a huge public party at his ancestral home, Lambton Park, complete with spitted ox and fireworks.

But like many a politician before and since, Anthony Lambton gradually reached the conclusion that his sexual needs could no longer be fulfilled in the marital bed. He began to look elsewhere, a course of action he was later to regret.

By 1973 he was openly visiting an attractive

26-year-old prostitute called Norma Levy, firstly at expensive hotels in London's West End and later at her own well-appointed flat in Maida Vale.

Norma's husband, Colin, knew all about her business and gave her his full backing. As a jobless cab driver who liked to spend freely on heavy drinking sessions, he had become accustomed to a healthy income. However, Levy was greedy, he wanted to make big money.

Sometimes Levy would spot his wife's clients coming out of the flat and wonder who they were and how much they were worth.

Slowly the germ of an idea grew into a full-blown plan. What if these men were both rich and famous? How much would photographs of them be worth?

Levy was not stupid enough to attempt blackmail; he knew only too well the risk of a long prison sentence.

But selling the story to the newspapers was another matter entirely. That was both legal and lucrative.

Levy decided his target would be the tall, well-spoken 'Mr Lucas', a customer who oozed wealth from the quality of his shirts and the cut of his suit. But how to find out his real name?

In the end, the client offered himself to Levy on a plate. Short of cash after one visit to Norma, he simply whipped out his cheque book and wrote her a £50 fee.

The cheque was signed Anthony Claud Frederick Lambton. It immediately identified him as parliamentary under-secretary at the Ministry of Defence, minister in charge of the Royal Air Force. Not only was Lambton famous, he was one of the wealthiest men in Britain.

With his prey out in the open, Levy now set about springing the trap.

He positioned a camera in Norma's bedroom wardrobe, installed a two-way mirror and concealed a microphone inside a teddy bear to pick up any juicy snippets of conversation.

The photographs showed a middle-aged man resting on a bed with two prostitutes and smoking a roll-your-own cigarette. It was unquestionably Lambton. The tape, meanwhile, included an admission that his lordship was a regular smoker of cannabis.

Triumphantly, Levy began hawking his 'scoop'. He started with Britain's biggest and most sensational Sunday newspaper, *The News of the World*, and arrived for a meeting with journalists expecting them to grill him thoroughly. But if he thought his story would drop like a bombshell, he was disappointed.

Reporters for *The News of the World* had been investigating Lambton for months following a tip-off that several senior politicians were involved with a ring of call girls.

There was little Levy could tell them that was new and after a few weeks he was told bluntly that there was no deal.

In an attempt to salvage something from the wreckage, Levy tried selling his story elsewhere in Fleet Street, with a price tag of £30,000. He also went to the West German magazine *Stern*, which showed great enthusiasm but refused to pay any money.

For *Stern* editors, free from the shackles of Britain's highly restrictive libel laws, the story was theirs for free. They prepared to published a colourful account of the scandal-tainted lifestyle of British MPs.

News of the magazine's plans spread like wildfire around Fleet Street. The journalists of *The News of the World*, distinctly uneasy at the prospect of losing their exclusive, decided they had to make Scotland Yard aware of their investigation. Suddenly the scandal reached boiling point.

On 21 May 1973, just as a disappointed Colin and Norma Levy headed for Spain and a secret hideaway, Lambton arrived at the offices of New Scotland Yard for an interview with two senior policeman: Deputy Assistant Commissioner Ernie Bond and Commander Bert Wickstead.

Lambton paced the floor nervously, his coat draped around his shoulders in the manner of some cloaked Gothic hero.

Yes, he knew Norma Levy. Yes, he had been to bed with her. She was 'a kind of prostitute'.

While his career was in tatters, Lambton was not yet admitting any offence. There was nothing illegal about paying for sex from a call girl. But the next question floored Lambton ...

"Have you taken drugs in her presence?" asked Bond.

Trapped, the minister made a full confession. Gone was the dismissive air of self confidence as he admitted the cigarette seen in the photographs was probably laced with cannabis.

Later he took the two policemen to his flat in London's St John's Wood and produced both cannabis resin and amphetamine tablets from a hidden cupboard. He knew he faced a criminal prosecution and the added disgrace of a public scandal.

"This is the end of my political career," he murmured to the officers. "I shall resign as soon as I return to my office."

The following day he issued a statement and took the opportunity to turn on those who had unmasked him. He declared:

"This is the sordid story. There has been no security risk and no blackmail and never at any time have I spoken of any aspect of my late job."

"All that has happened is that some sneak pimp has seen an opportunity of making money by the sale of the story and secret photographs to papers at home and abroad."

"My own feelings may be imagined but I have no excuses whatsoever to make. I behaved with credulous stupidity."

JOHN VASSALL

In the early 60s the British security service, MI5, prided itself on its supposed ability to prevent penetration by Soviet intelligence. Senior 'molecatchers' had devised a system of positive vetting which, they believed, made it impossible for a double agent to be planted at any senior level within the organisation. Whatever else the Reds might use to undermine Britain during the Cold War, the risk of traitors spilling secrets was felt to be minor.

It was with some scepticism then that the British Embassy in Washington received a 'most urgent' call from colleagues at the US Central Intelligence Agency.

The Royal Navy's operations role within the North Atlantic Treaty Organisation had been betrayed to the Soviets. The traitor was working in the heart of Whitehall and had to be stopped before NATO's key Atlantic warfare strategy was betrayed. Such was the urgency that the CIA officer responsible decided there was no time for a face-to-face meeting.

As he put the phone down he felt relief that MI5 would soon be on the case.

However, the British reaction over the next few days left the Americans bewildered and frustrated. Rather than preparing a counter-intelligence coup, MI5 sniffily responded that the information was most unlikely to be accurate. The episode was, they were convinced, an attempt by the Soviets to dupe the West into a wild goose chase.

The aim would be to occupy the time of British case officers who could otherwise be chasing genuine spies. Moreover, MI5 believed that any security witch-hunt would serve only to sap the morale of many conscientious and hard-working civil servants.

In the months ahead, this woefully smug stance would lead to incalculable damage to Anglo-US intelligence relations and send MI5's reputation to rock bottom. It still stands out as one of the great post-war botch-ups by the service.

The CIA's source was KGB defector Anatoli Golytsin, who had swapped sides at Christmas 1961. He had already pointed to a massive spying web in France and had unmasked a top Canadian Foreign Office official as a committed KGB agent.

Yet when the men from MI5 flew out in March 1962 to interview him they remained unconvinced of his account that a spy had penetrated the Admiralty. They wondered whether Golytsin was still a KGB agent who had 'defected' so that he could spread dis-information amongst the Western intelligence agencies.

Positive vetting, they pointed out to the CIA, involved exhaustive checks of a subject's personal life and his ideological background. They could not believe the system had failed in this case. Eventually however, in deference to the Americans, they agreed to launch an investigation.

Enquiries rumbled on for five months without success. Then the CIA team came up with another breakthrough.

A Soviet United Nations official who had been 'turned' was talking about a highly-placed British mole.

The guilty officer was a homosexual who had been blackmailed by the KGB while serving as a diplomat at Britain's Moscow agency. One man's name was instantly in the frame.

John Vassall, 38, was a former assistant private secretary to the Civil Lord of the Admiralty. He had been a naval attaché's clerk in Moscow from 1954 to 1956 and, since moving to his new job in the Fleet Section of Military Branch II at the Admiralty, he had processed and filed hundreds of top secret papers.

At last the MI5 machine was moving. Staff arranged to temporarily move in to a flat at London's exclusive Dolphin Square riverside development – next door to the bachelor pad owned by Vassall.

He was kept under observation for several days until his movements were established. Then one morning, while he was at his desk, the professional spycatchers slipped the lock on his front door and searched the flat from top to bottom.

They had been trained in the art of discovering hidey holes and it didn't take them long to find Vassall's.

A specially-doctored bookcase contained a miniature Exacta camera with rolls of film showing pictures of classified material.

The waiting game was over and on 12 September 1962 Vassall was picked up by police from the Special Branch as he left work and charged with espionage.

He cracked immediately and it was with a strong sense of relief that he began telling his interrogators how the KGB had turned him. It had started in Moscow, where the young Vassall felt out of place in the company of fellow embassy officers.

He developed a friendship with a good-looking Russian man called Mikhailski and they began an intimate sexual relationship. Vassall realised the implications of what he was doing but convinced himself there was no harm in it. He was always careful what he said to his young lover.

It was of course the classic 'honey-trap'

beloved by thriller writers. Mikhailski was a KGB officer who expertly lured Vassall into a situation in which he rapidly lost control.

He began by accompanying the Briton to the theatre, the ballet and some of Moscow's most exclusive restaurants.

And when a senior embassy colleague warned Vassall about such flagrant socialising it was Mikhailski who suggested they be more discreet. One weekend he floated the idea of attending a private party at the Hotel Berlin.

There Vassall drank himself almost to a stupor. He took part in an all-male orgy, indulging in a number of highly explicit sex acts which were faithfully captured on film by one of the KGB officers present.

When he sobered up Vassall agonized over whether he should tell his embassy colleagues what he'd done.

He decided against it. At that time, homo-sexuality was an offence in Britain, and in the Soviet Union it was a serious crime.

Some months later the KGB sprung the honey trap. They established that Vassall had been allocated a new job at the Admiralty in London, a job where he would have access to some of the Navy's most sensitive operational secrets. It was the perfect role in which to run a double-agent.

The hapless Vassall was invited to a private

Moscow apartment where the photographs were shown to him.

The senior KGB man present told him he had two choices. Either he could be arrested as a homosexual and forced to serve a hard, lengthy imprisonment in a Soviet jail. Or he could agree to continue meeting a KGB officer called Gregory in London – a man he recognised from the fateful orgy – and pass on interesting information. Failure to comply would automatically mean his exposure to his superiors.

By now Vassall was in a whirl of confusion and under enormous stress.

Yet it would still not have been too late to go to his own seniors and confess. Had he done so, he might have been welcomed with open arms because MI5 rarely had such an opportunity to disrupt Soviet intelligence gathering. Playing Vassall as a turned double-agent would have allowed them to mislead the Soviets over the Navy's true North Atlantic mandate.

It was not to be. Vassall began to pass intelligence to Gregory at a series of clandestine meetings in Underground stations and telephone kiosks. By the time the CIA stemmed the flow the Royal Navy was seriously compromised.

Vassall was given an eighteen-year jail sentence, later reduced to ten with parole.

His case brought about a government inquiry

into MI5's internal security, at which the service had to admit that its method of positive vetting had been an unmitigated disaster. Incredibly, two of Vassall's character references had been old ladies who had made clear his reluctance to socialise with the opposite sex. Despite this very obvious signal, Vassall achieved a top-level security clearance.

THE KENNEDYS

Americans' fascination for the British Royal Family almost surpasses that of the British themselves. It is a strange preoccupation for a nation that since its birth has constitutionally shunned such an institution. Whatever the reason, it does help explain why the United States of America created its own 'royals' where none could possibly exist. The name of this dynasty? The Kennedys.

Yet this multimillion-dollar dynasty has been involved in scandal since it first arrived on the world stage. And the golden 'First Family' has not thrown off its odour to this day.

The power of the Kennedy family was founded on crime. In the Twenties, gangsters like Al Capone built their power and reputation on bootlegging – smuggling booze to illicit drinking dens to beat the US government's Prohibition – and Joseph Kennedy Sr followed them.

The young Joe ploughed the profits into the Stock Market and property. He was a multimillionaire by the age of 35, and he married heiress Rose Fitzgerald, daughter of the mayor of Boston.

She was a strict disciplinarian but, after raising nine children and finding that scandal beset most of them, she was forced to admit:

"When I think of our past I try to dwell on the good times and not to be haunted by the bad. There have been moments awesome in their horror."

On another occasion she said: "God never sends his cross heavier than we can bear."

They were brave words, given that she often to stifle her own at her husband's indiscretions. Throughout their marriage, Rose had to suffer silently as her husband enjoyed a string of affairs, the most notorious of which was with actress Gloria Swanson.

He used to tell his mistresses: "Make love with me and you'll never want to make love with anyone else.

Joseph Kennedy was also politically indiscreet. When he was appointed Ambassador to Britain in the run-up to World War II, he displayed his strong Irish sympathies and fought to keep the US out of the conflict.

He was recalled ignominiously after telling a newspaper:

"Democracy is finished here in Britain. If the US gets into the war with England, we will be left holding the bag."

The old man's sons inherited his Irish loyalties. Similarly, they inherited his love of power, as was epitomised by the political careers of John,

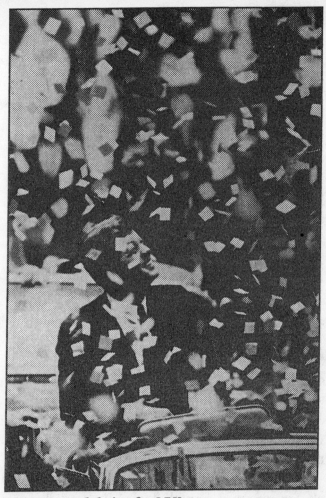

Ticker-tape adulation for J.F.K.

Robert and Edward. Unfortunately, they also inherited his sexual appetites outside marriage.

After the shock of the assassination of John F. Kennedy, in Dallas in 1963, had subsided, reports began to emerge of his lifelong philandering ....

One of his earliest indiscretions was as a 24-year-old naval intelligence officer during World War II when he fell in love with ex-Miss Denmark Inga Fejos. Unfortunately, she was reputed to have been a spy working for the Nazis. Joe Kennedy Sr used his influence to end the affair by having his son transferred to a torpedo boat in the Pacific. The young naval officer is quoted as saying: "They shipped my ass out of town to break us up."

Despite his marriage to the beautiful Jacqueline Bouvier in 1953, the number of his mistresses ran into triple figures. And Kennedy was a womaniser who pursued his pleasures with little heed for national security.

He shocked British Prime Minister Harold Macmillan when, during the 1962 summit in Nassau, he told him: "I get severe headaches when I go too long without a woman."

He absented himself for an hour with two female members of his personal retinue, and returned to tell the British Premier: "My headache's gone now."

Back home at the White House he would take

advantage of Jacqueline's absences by disporting himself naked around the swimming pool with one or more young ladies. Regular duties of his security staff included searching bedding for blonde hairs and carpets for hairpins. On one occasion they failed to detect a pair of woman's panties in the marital bedroom. Upon discovering them, Jackie handed them to her husband, saying simply: "They're not my size."

Thomas C. Reeves, in his book *A Question Of Character: A Life Of John F. Kennedy*, described a sex session that supposedly took place on the very night of the President's inauguration and the use of a prostitute on the night of Kennedy's vital television confrontation with presidential rival Richard Nixon.

Once in office, according to Reeves, Kennedy seduced a new White House secretary by the name of Pamela Turnure. JFK advised his wife to hire Turnure so that she would be close at hand when he needed her.

Jackie must have been suspicious at the time because she questioned Jack's choice of secretary, the girl being young and pretty but wholly unqualified for the job.

In another book, aptly titled *Presidential Passions*, author Michael John Sullivan revealed a further twist to the tale of JFK and the hiring of his wife's secretary.

Sullivan said that Jack soon lost interest in Pam Turnure and began sleeping with Washington socialite Mary Pinchot Meyer, a 'friend' of Jackie. The affair began in 1962 and continued through about 30 visits to the White House, during one of which they retired to a bedroom with six marijuana joints. During their wild lovemaking, Jack confided to her that he was chairing a conference on drug abuse in a few days time.

The affair with Meyer continued right up until JFK's assassination. Less than a year after his death, Mary was herself shot dead while strolling in broad daylight near her home. The killer was never caught and no motive was ever discovered for the mysterious murder.

Most of Kennedy's affairs were short term, most lasting only an hour or so. Others, however, were of greater importance to him – and of the gravest worry to his secret service protectors. Among these was his love affair with the most feted beauty in the world: movie star Marilyn Monroe.

JFK was introduced to Marilyn by his brother-in-law Peter Lawford. Actor Lawford, who had married Jack's sister Pat, had a Los Angeles beachfront home which was used as a Californian base both by Jack and his brother Robert, the US Attorney General. Both of them had affairs with Marilyn Monroe ...

The actress was dreadfully unstable at this time, and even to have encouraged her into clandestine friendships would have been cruel beyond belief. Yet both the President and his brother cynically toyed with her then harshly ditched her when she became too much of a nuisance to them.

Their treatment of her had the most tragic consequences and prompted one of the most ferocious cover-ups in political history.

At the height of her affair with Jack, Marilyn even travelled in disguise on the presidential aircraft US One.

She was there at his side at his 45th birthday party in Madison Square Gardens when she sang a shaky *Happy Birthday To You*. But as her mental state deteriorated and she turned increasingly to drink and drugs, Marilyn was snubbed by the Kennedy brothers. The word went out from the White House that she was no longer to contact her ex-lovers.

On 5 August 1962 Marilyn was found dead at her Los Angeles home – and rumours of her affairs with Jack and Bobby Kennedy began to sweep Hollywood.

Theories that she had been silenced grew stronger.

It was said that her house had been bugged by

the Attorney General, by the FBI or even by Jimmy Hoffa, head of the Mafia-linked Teamsters Union, who was seeking incriminating evidence against his arch-enemy Robert Kennedy.

It was said that she had had an abortion shortly before her death and that the father could have been Bobby.

It was certainly the fact that Marilyn had tried to contact him at the Justice Department in Washington several times in the weeks before her death. But her 'nuisance' calls had not been put through.

Several authors, including the renowned Norman Mailer, advanced the theory that Marilyn had been murdered by secret service agents to protect the Kennedy brothers from worldwide disgrace.

A bizarre twist to this theory came twenty years later in a book *Mafia Kingpin* by reformed criminal Ronald 'Sonny' Gibson. He said that while working for the mobsters he had learned of a unique deal between the FBI and the Mafia.

FBI chief J. Edgar Hoover had been furious with Marilyn over her embarrassing affairs with leading politicians and had agreed to turn a blind eye to her removal.

The Mafia therefore ordered hitmen to bump off the star in order to repay old favours done for them by the FBI.

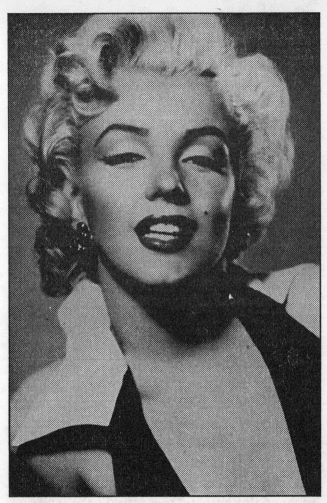

Marilyn Monroe ... said to be the lover of two Kennedy brothers.

If such theories seemed far-fetched, they were no wilder than the truth itself: that the most powerful man in the world (and his brother) had been having a clandestine affair with the most popular film star ever known! And no wilder than the fact that, at another stage of his licentious life, the President was having an affair with a Mafia gangster's moll.

Sam Giancana was one of the most powerful Mafia godfathers in the US. His lover was Judith Campbell Exner. In February 1960 JFK, then a Massachusetts senator, attended a party thrown by his friend and political supporter Frank Sinatra.

There Jack was introduced to the glamorous Judith and immediately set about wooing her to his bed. He succeeded, and for two years the couple were lovers.

In her autobiography *My Story*, the dark-haired, blue-eyed beauty spoke of passionate meetings, of Kennedy's chronic back pains and the sexual problems it caused him, of his desire for a three-in-a-bed romp (and her refusal) and how their affair ended in 1962 when they parted without bitterness, because of the risks of discovery and disgrace.

Certainly Judith Campbell Exner visited the White House on many occasions. Certainly she met JFK not only in Washington but in Chicago,

Los Angeles and Palm Beach. She may even, as she claimed, have been Kennedy's link with the Mafia, regularly carrying sealed packages between White House aides and her mob mate Giancana.

There is no proof, however, that she arranged ten meetings between Giancana and Kennedy, at least one of them being about the attempted overthrow of Cuban dictator Fidel Castro.

The Exner-Kennedy affair came to light when a Senate select committee on intelligence affairs began investigating links between the CIA and attempts on Castro's life.

These inquiries led to Giancana, then to Exner, and thence to Jack Kennedy. The White House telephone log revealed 70 calls were made between the President and Exner in a 54-week period of 1961 and 1962. Some were between the White House and The Oak Park, Illinois, home of Sam Giancana.

In her book, Exner 'revealed' that, while visiting the White House, she had noted many phone calls to the President from FBI chief Hoover. What she probably did not know was that many of them were warnings from Hoover that his liaison with the gangster's moll could lay him open to blackmail – or become so public that it would destroy him anyway.

Also in her book, Exner 'revealed' that in the

early days of her affair with Kennedy, his younger brother, Edward, also tried to date her. She turned him down. This small revelation caused no surprise at all when the American public read Judith's book. For Teddy Kennedy was already known as a womaniser. Although it was not so much his dalliances as his deception – over the drowning of a girl in his car at Chappaquiddick Island – which muddied his career.

ROMAN POLANSKI

Film director Roman Polanski had seen the ultimate horrors of war at first hand. Born into a Jewish family in 1933, his parents were removed by the Nazis and his mother died in Auschwitz concentration camp. His experiences were often mirrored in his early, violent movies, particularly *Knife In The Water*, *Repulsion* and *Rosemary's Baby*. Psychiatrists claimed later that his traumatic childhood experiences in Nazi-occupied Cracow, Poland, were the cause not only of some of the more sickening scenes in his films but for the scandals that almost wrecked his life.

In 1968 *Rosemary's Baby* was released to acclaim, and to some adverse criticism because of its voyeuristic violence.

By now a resident of California, Polanski flew to London to marry the beautiful, 26-year-old actress Sharon Tate, whom he had starred in one of his earlier movies, the horror spoof *Dance Of The Vampires*. Hollywood movie moguls hoped that Polanski, who had gained notoriety for his free-spirited lifestyle through the drug-taking, sexually permissive sixties, would now lead a more settled existence.

The friends he gathered around him back in

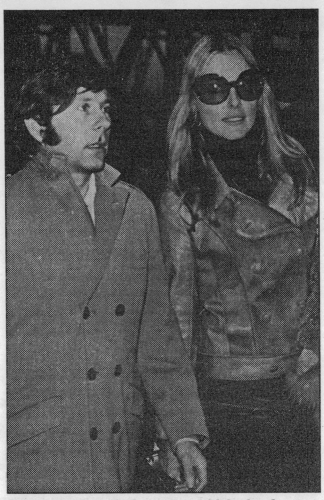

Brutally butchered: Sharon Tate with husband
Roman Polanski.

Los Angeles, however, were not free of the taint of drugs and promiscuity.

In February 1969 Roman and Sharon moved into a mansion in Cielo Drive, Benedict Canyon, a house previously occupied by Doris Day's son, Terry Melcher. The following month a scruffy hippy-style character arrived at the gate and was turned away. He was the evil cult leader Charles Manson.

Manson did not call again – but four of his followers did. Shortly before dawn on 9 August 1969, while Polanski was away in London working on a screenplay, the four 'Angels Of Death' entered the grounds of the house in Cielo Drive, where Sharon Tate and some of the Polanskis' friends had been carousing, some of them in a state of drug-induced euphoria.

Within a couple of hours, they had completed their grisly task – and five people lay dead in an orgy of butchery. The scene these Angels of Death left behind them turned the stomachs of even the most hardened of Los Angeles cops.

When police arrived on the scene, they found the body of Steven Parent, the eighteen-year-old guest of the house's caretaker, slumped in his car in the driveway. Parent had encountered the raiders as he drove from the house, had been flagged down and shot four times.

The body of Abigail Folger, heiress to a coffee

fortune, was found lying on the lawn. She had been cut to pieces as she tried to flee. The other bodies were found in the house.

Polanski's compatriot, Polish film director Voytek Frykowski, was found battered almost beyond recognition. He had awoken from a drugged sleep to find the killers standing over him. Hit with a club, he had then been finished off with six thrusts of a knife. Hollywood hair stylist Jay Sebring had been stabbed then dispatched with a gunshot.

The most sickening sight, however, was the pathetic body of beautiful Sharon Tate. The actress, eight months pregnant, had suffered sixteen stab wounds. Her unborn baby boy died along with her.

The perpetrators of this vile crime (three women and one man who, along with Manson himself, were later convicted of the slaughter) had all been fired up with drugs for their orgy of blood-letting.

The American public were disgusted – but when they learned that drugs had also been regularly taken within the house of horror, the reaction changed. Irrationally, Polanski himself was blamed for being part of Hollywood's hippy culture.

"You can hear the toilets flushing all over Beverly Hills," said one observer referring to the hasty end of the Sixties drug culture.

After the horrors of Cielo Drive and the recriminations that followed, Polanski, if anything, grew even wilder. His great friend was the actor Jack Nicholson and the pair were known for their partying and womanising. It was at Nicholson's Los Angeles home that Polanski's scandalous lifestyle finally caught up with him – and finally caught him out.

Polanski had invited a thirteen-year-old girl to pose for him for a magazine study of youthful beauty. The photo shoot began in Nicholson's swimming pool, continued with the consumption of a bottle of champagne, and ended with the girl half-naked in the jacuzzi.

It was said later that the girl, who was asthmatic, at some stage suffered an attack and that Polanski gave her a Quaalude tranquilliser, which is also believed to have properties as a 'love drug'. The girl later fell asleep on a bed – but only after, it was alleged, the film director had had sex with her.

In a statement later made to police, the girl said she phoned her mother (herself an ex-lover of Polanski) to ask permission to go to bed with the director; the mother 'reluctantly' agreed.

Roman Polanski's night with the naked teenager ended when Jack Nicholson's girlfriend, Angelica Huston, returned home unexpectedly, realised what was going on and threw the pair out of the house.

When the girl returned to her own home, she told her boyfriend and sister of the night's events. Together they tackled her mother, who seemingly changed her mind about her daughter's libertarian lifestyle, and they phoned the police. Polanski was arrested in a room at the Beverly Wilshire Hotel. The girl was also taken into custody. Jack Nicholson's house was then searched, a small quantity of drugs found, and Angelica Huston was charged with possession.

The result was that Polanski was indicted by a Grand Jury on six counts:

1. Furnishing a controlled substance to a minor.

2. Committing a lewd and lascivious act on a thirteen-year-old child.

3. Unlawful sexual intercourse.

4. Rape by use of drugs, including Quaalude and alcohol.

5. Perversion, including copulating in the mouth with the sexual organ of the child.

6. Sodomy.

Plea bargaining began and Polanski pleaded guilty to the third count, the least serious of the charges: Unlawful sexual intercourse.

Polanski's lawyer also offered the court that the director would found a theatre arts school for

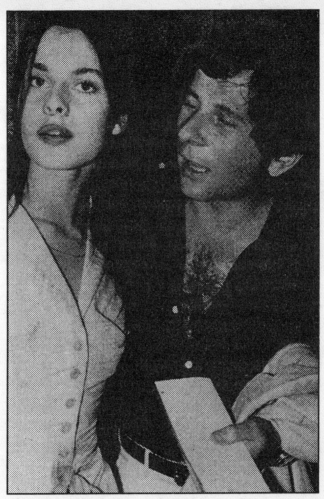

After his wife's death, Polanski fell for starlet
Nastassia Kinski.

poor children. The child's parents were mollified but the judge was not.

Judge Lawrence J. Rittenband ruled:

"Although the prosecutrix was not an inexperienced girl, this is of course not a licence to the defendant, a man of the world in his forties, to engage in an act of unlawful sexual intercourse with her."

"The law was designed for the protection of females under the age of eighteen years, and it is no defence to such a charge that the female might not have resisted the act."

Polanski was ordered to spend 90 days undergoing psychiatric and other tests at a state centre, along with other inmates he disdainfully dismissed as "the scum of society."

After that he was again to face the judge to receive his full sentence. Polanski served out only part of his 90 days of tests before getting permission to make a series of trips to Paris to work on other movies. He confidently anticipated a deal whereby he would eventually walk from court scot-free.

The judge had other ideas, however. Early in 1978 Judge Rittenband became infuriated by the roaming director's flaunting of his love affair with sixteen-year-old starlet Nastassia Kinski throughout the preparations for the case. Polanski's lawyers warned him to expect some sort of custodial sentence - and he decided to flee the US. Since he had already travelled several times from Los Angeles to France without being stopped by the authorities, Polanski quietly boarded a night flight to Paris on 31 January 1978. There, safe from extradition, he determined never to return to his adoptive country. Disgusted, Judge Rittenband transferred the case to another judge. The papers were filed away to gather dust.

JEREMY THORPE

Illicit sex, blackmail, allegations of attempted murder, secret service plots ... the Jeremy Thorpe case had all the ingredients of the political scandal of the century.

When John Jeremy Thorpe, MP, lawyer, Privy Councillor and former leader of the Liberal Party, faced a court accused of inciting three men who stood in the dock alongside him to murder a former male model with whom he was alleged to have had an affair, it was the biggest scandal since the John Profumo/Christine Keeler case, when the War Minister had been dragged down in a morass of sleaze, prostitution and spy stories.

Thorpe, born 29 April 1929, the son of a well-to-do Tory MP, was destined to be a high-flier. He was educated at Eton and Oxford University, where he became president of the Oxford Union, the springboard for many a successful political career.

He was called to the bar in 1954, but he opted for politics and in 1959 was narrowly elected the Liberal Party's Member of Parliament for North Devon.

A born orator, his wit and style carried him to ever greater success. In seven years, he was leader of his party and, in the political situation of the

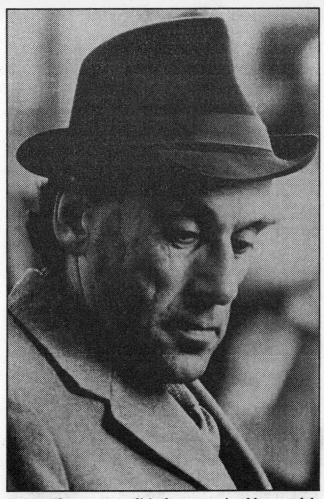

Jeremy Thorpe ... a political career ruined by scandal.

day, a possible Cabinet minister in a coalition government.

Throughout his parliamentary career, however, a time bomb was ticking away remorselessly. It was to explode in his face at the Old Bailey in May 1979 and precipitate a downfall even more spectacular than his meteoric rise.

Thorpe's affected mannerisms and style had not gone unnoticed, and in 1960 a routine check by the security services had concluded that he had homosexual tendencies, still a criminal activity at the time. The report was filed and forgotten.

It was to be a momentous year for the young MP. On a visit to an Oxfordshire riding school, he came face to face with his nemesis: Norman Josiffe, later known as Norman Scott.

Josiffe, eleven years Thorpe's junior, was the emotionally disturbed child of a broken marriage, on probation for larceny. The two men struck up a friendship, and the MP told him to get in contact if he ever needed help. It was an offer he was to regret.

A year later, after an unsuccessful suicide bid, Josiffe remembered his important friend, and on 8 November 1961 the two met at the House of Commons, after which Thorpe offered to put the young man up at his mother's home in Oxted, Surrey.

It was there, according to Josiffe, that their

affair began. Thorpe allegedly gave Josiffe a copy of James Baldwin's novel, *Giovanni's Room*, and later knocked on his door and entered, wearing a dressing gown.

According to Josiffe: "He said I looked liked a frightened rabbit. He hugged me, called me 'poor bunny' and got into bed with me."

Giving evidence later, he said Thorpe then sodomised him. He claimed he did not enjoy the experience, but "bit the pillow and tried not to scream." His version of events was steadfastly denied by Thorpe.

In any case, the friendship continued. Thorpe helped Josiffe find a job. When Josiffe was accused of stealing a coat, Thorpe again came to the rescue, insisting that police interview Josiffe in his office because he was the young man's guardian.

When Josiffe went to work on a farm in Somerset, Thorpe wrote him affectionate letters, one of which ended with the curiously coded message: "Bunnies can (and will) go to France."

When he lost that job, however, Thorpe refused to help him further and Josiffe started making threats against his powerful mentor. When this came to the ears of police in December 1962, he was taken in for questioning and again poured out his allegations of an affair with Thorpe. Though they took the 'Bunnies' letter, the

Chelsea police did not follow up the allegations. This was due to a lack of any hard evidence.

Thorpe had a brief respite from the demands and threats when Josiffe sought work abroad, first in Ireland then in Switzerland. But again, when these jobs ended in failure, he returned to Britain and the claims against the politician were renewed. Thorpe asked a fellow Liberal MP to be his go-between with Josiffe. Peter Bessell was another potential high-flier, though later he was to emerge as a shady businessman, forced to leave the country for a time to escape creditors. Bessell was to be Thorpe's ally in stopping Josiffe. When that failed, he was to be the fall guy.

Whatever hold Josiffe had over the MP became all the more politically dangerous in January 1967 when Thorpe succeeded Jo Grimond as leader of the Liberal Party. At this stage, according to prosecuting lawyers a decade later, the politician determined to have his former lover killed ...

In a conversation with Bessell, Thorpe allegedly said: "We have got to get rid of him."

Bessell asked: "Are you suggesting killing him off?"

Thorpe allegedly replied: "Yes."

In 1969, Thorpe must have felt a surge of relief when Josiffe, having taken up modelling and now calling himself Scott, got married. For Thorpe, himself married to a wealthy, elegant and supportive wife, the relief was short-lived. Scott's wife sued for divorce in the autumn of 1970 when he admitted sleeping with a boyfriend.

Emotionally disturbed, Scott began telling journalists about his illicit relationship with a leading politician. He also threatened to reveal incriminating letters, this time written to him by Bessell on Thorpe's behalf.

It was then that a businessman friend, David Holmes, was dispatched to pay him £2,500. Scott moved to a cottage on Exmoor and began to drink heavily and to take drugs.

Here he was contacted by a man calling himself 'Keene', who warned him that his life was in danger from a killer hired in Canada. Scott agreed to meet the contact in the village of Combe Martin on 24 October 1975. He took his Great Dane, Rinka, along.

Keene, whose real name was Andrew Newton, an airline pilot, put Scott at his ease and the two drove off together.

On a lonely stretch of moorland road, Newton stopped the car on a pretext and the two men got out. The next thing Scott remembered was staring into the barrel of a gun in the hand of his new-found 'friend'.

The dog was barking excitedly. "This is it," said Newton – and shot the dog. Turning to Scott he allegedly said: "It's your turn now." He pulled the trigger but the gun apparently jammed. Newton jumped into the car and drove away.

A passing motorist later picked up Scott and police quickly traced Newton, whose defence was that he was being blackmailed by Scott and had shot the dog in order to frighten him off. He was jailed for two years and served a little more than half.

Scott was not scared off, however, and when he found himself in court on a charge of defrauding the Social Security Department, Jeremy Thorpe's nightmare came true ...

Scott had never been able to prove a homosexual liaison, so he could have been prosecuted for libel if any newspaper were to have printed his story (homosexuality was no longer a crime, but it still carried a stigma). But in a court of law, he could make his accusations under 'privilege'.

Thus it was that, in a court case in which he was charged with defrauding the piffling sum of £58.40, Scott blurted out that he was being hounded because of a relationship with Thorpe. The story was out.

Thorpe immediately denied the affair and told his political colleagues that Scott was a blackmailer and that his real target was Peter Bessell, who had been having an affair with his secretary. Bessell was even persuaded to write a letter backing this up, on the understanding that it would be published only as a last resort. In fact it was leaked to the press almost immediately. Bessell later moved to California to escape creditors. From there, he supported an anti-Thorpe movement within the Liberal Party.

The then Labour Prime Minister, Harold Wilson, added a new dimension to the scandal when he suggested that the South African security services had been at work to smear Thorpe, who was an outspoken opponent of apartheid. Not that this helped Thorpe, as journalists began probing ever deeper.

On 10 May 1976 Jeremy Thorpe was forced to resign as party leader. For a year the scandal lay dormant and Thorpe's political career continued.

In April 1977, however, Newton came out of jail and decided that someone should pay for his year's incarceration. He touted his secrets to the London Evening News, which paid him £3,000 for his story, run that October under the headline 'I Was Hired To Kill Scott'.

The scandal burst forth again. Newspapers were full of 'the South Wales Connection': the allegation that hitman Newton had been in the pay of Port Talbot businessmen John Le Mesurier and George Deakin. A third alleged backer, David Holmes, was also being investigated. In August

1978 warrants were issued for the arrest of all three, along with Thorpe, on charges of conspiracy to murder. Thorpe was additionally charged with incitement to murder. All denied the charges.

The foursome appeared at the Old Bailey on 8 May 1979, where an astonishing story of sexual scandal and criminal intrigue was expounded in the measured tones of the English legal profession.

The prosecution made much of the seduction of Scott and claimed that the affair had continued for a considerable time. Bessell told of the 'kill Scott' conversation and alleged that Holmes had been asked by Thorpe to poison Scott and dump his body in a disused tin mine shaft.

The court heard that Holmes had approached Le Mesurier and Deakin for help in 'frightening off a blackmailer'. Deakin sought the help of a Cardiff printer, David Miller, who in turn recommended Newton. Newton, although he claimed he had no intention of killing Scott, had been paid £5,000 by Miller and Le Mesurier on his release from jail.

It was further alleged that this money had been siphoned off from party funds. Things looked black for Thorpe when the prosecution rested.

George Carman QC, for the defence, set about discrediting the witnesses. Bessell was forced to admit that he had a contract with a newspaper to sell his story. The price would be £50,000 if Thorpe were convicted, £25,000 if he were acquitted. Bessell's evidence was further put into question when Carman referred to a plot by Bessell to defraud a wealthy Liberal Party benefactor of £500,000, and to Bessell's admission that he had left the country in 1974 to escape creditors.

Scott, too, was forced to admit that even before his House of Commons meeting with Thorpe, he had been boasting of having an affair with him. The inference was that he had intended the affair to happen – so the seduction was a myth. Scott was made to look like a neurotic, hounding an innocent man out of malice.

Newton fared no better, being forced to admit that he had lied under oath at his original trial for shooting Scott's dog.

Of the accused, only Deakin chose to go into the witness box. He said he had merely helped find someone to frighten a blackmailer. He neither knew, nor cared, who was the victim.

Summing up, Mr Justice Cantley pointed out that Bessell's allegations of the 'kill Scott' conversation were uncorroborated and described Scott as a "hysterical, warped personality, an accomplished liar and a crook." The jury took two days to acquit all four accused.

Thorpe, then, was innocent – but his battle to retain his political power and prestige was already in vain.

Just four days before the Old Bailey trial had begun, a General Election had taken place, called by the new Labour Prime Minister, James Callaghan. Arrogantly and against the advice of colleagues, Thorpe had decided to fight for his North Devon seat. On 3 May 1979, twenty years after winning the seat, Thorpe saw his 7,000 majority overturned and the Tories sweep in by 8,473 votes.

Jeremy Thorpe's downfall was complete.

JOYCE MCKINNEY

It began on 15 September 1977 with a brief statement from Scotland Yard. Nothing too dramatic, but enough to arouse the curiosity of a few seasoned crime reporters. A young Mormon missionary, said the Yard, had vanished "in most unusual circumstances". The spokesman added: "We cannot rule out the possibility that he has been abducted."

Probing deeper, the journalists discovered that the American missionary's name was Kirk Anderson, aged 21, from Salt Lake City. He had apparently received a call from a man called Bob Bosler, who had expressed an interest in turning to Anderson's faith.

The young priest had met Bosler at the Mormon church in East Ewell, Surrey, and joined him and a friend to show them the milelong route to the church offices. None of the three had been seen since.

So far, the story was intriguing, though hardly front page news. Within hours, however, new revelations had Fleet Street's editors champing at the bit.

Salt Lake City police wired Scotland Yard to warn that before visiting Britain Anderson had suffered persistent harassment from a woman

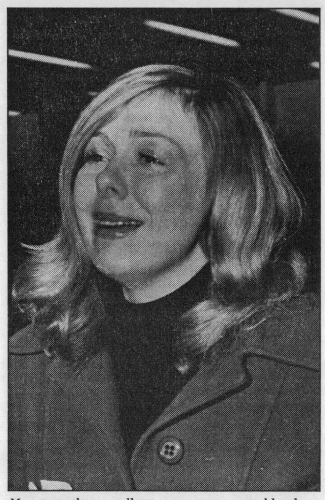

Man-trap: the sexually outrageous runaway blonde
Joyce McKinney.

who seemed mentally unstable. Even more fascinating was the suggestion from Mormon Church officials that he had been kidnapped because he 'scorned a wealthy woman's love'.

It appeared the woman concerned had hired a small army of private detectives to pursue him across America. The trip to Britain was his way of escaping her.

Within three days, Kirk Anderson turned up and confirmed that the story was true. The woman and two accomplices had kept him handcuffed and manacled for 72 hours in a remote cottage. Detective Chief Superintendent Hucklesby, head of the CID 'Z' Division, announced that police were searching for two Americans travelling as man and wife. One was Keith Joseph May, alias Bob Bosler, alias Paul Van Deusen, aged 24. The other was Joyce McKinney, alias Cathy Vaughn Bare, alias Heidi Krazler, aged 27. She had long blonde hair and a strong southern accent.

Hucklesby was asked by journalists if it would be right to describe McKinney as attractive? "Oh yes," he replied. "Very."

Later that same day the two suspects were picked up by police in the West Country driving along the A30. Officers had also discovered the secluded holiday cottage near Okehampton, Devon, where Anderson claimed he had been held in chains.

There were already rumours coming out of Devon that 'unusual discoveries' at the cottage had left the local police in stitches.

Understandably, Hucklesby found himself swamped with questions from the curious media pack. Off the record, he admitted that the Devon and Cornwall Constabulary had found 'certain equipment' at the cottage. "I can't go into details," he quipped, "but I'll tell you what. I've never been lucky enough to have anything like that happen to me."

On 22 September McKinney, described as a 'former beauty queen', and Keith May, a trainee architect, appeared in court accused of forcibly abducting and imprisoning Kirk Anderson and possessing an imitation .38 revolver with intent to commit an offence. The 'Sex In Chains' scandal was well underway.

At her next appearance the following week, Joyce – or Joy as she preferred to be known – showed she could milk publicity with the best of them. As the black maria van drew up outside Epsom magistrates court, she managed to fling four notes at the waiting pressmen.

They read: "Please tell the truth. My reputation is at stake!", "He had sex with me for four days.", "Please get the truth to the public. He made it look like kidnapping." and "Ask

Christians to pray for me."

There then ensued a battle as Joyce, wearing a flimsy cheesecloth outfit with loose neckline, tried to make a dash towards the reporters. Police restrained her but in the melee she managed to reveal her ample breasts to photographers. Clearly, McKinney was in no mood to let British justice take its normal course.

Over the next few weeks the police became more and more baffled by the bizarre case. Not least was Joyce McKinney's claim that, far from locking the missionary up in a Devon love-nest for four days, she, May and Anderson had twice been out shopping and dining together in London's West End.

The court committal hearing opened on 23 November with prosecutor Neil Dennison QC explaining how McKinney had developed a 'consuming desire' for Anderson when they first met in Provo, Utah. They had sex but as this was contrary to Mormon beliefs, Anderson later told her the relationship was over.

She refused to accept his decision, blaming the doctrine of his church. And so her epic attempt to pursue and seduce him began. When the trail led to England McKinney and May – a man described as her friend and mentor – hatched a plot to kidnap the missionary at gunpoint and drive him to Devon.

In the witness box, Kirk Anderson took up the story. He told how he had been chained spreadeagled to the four corners of the bed, after which McKinney ripped off his pyjamas, performed oral sex on him to arouse him and then proceeded to full intercourse. Later they had two further sessions of lovemaking.

Anderson went on: "She said she was going to get what she wanted, whether I wanted to or not. She said she might keep me there for another month or so until she missed her period."

McKinney's counsel, Stuart Elgrod, was unimpressed. Elgrod: "I am suggesting that at no stage were you ever tied up in that cottage except for the purpose of sex games."

Anderson: "No, no, that's wrong."

Elgrod: "The next day you were joking about it. You were completely unfettered."

Anderson: "I was bolted in."

Elgrod: "You didn't even try to escape?"

Anderson: "No, I knew I was going back soon anyway."

The case was adjourned and lawyers from both sides decamped to consider strategy. It certainly didn't look good for the prosecution. Anderson had admitted asking McKinney to rub his back.

He also agreed that he had thrown his so-called jailer across the bed in a fit of pique. Then there was the trip to London during his 'confinement' when he, McKinney and May had lunched at the Hard Rock Cafe. It hardly sounded like the experience of a man captured and held against his will.

McKinney was now spilling out her side of the story to police. She told how she and Anderson had enjoyed a three-year relationship in which he had made much of the running. How she had stocked up on his favourite food at the Devon cottage. How she bought his blue pyjamas, complete with name tag, and packed herself see-through nighties. And how she even remembered to bring the quilt on which she and Kirk first had sex.

She had dreamed up the bondage game, she said, after studying the books of Dr Alex Comfort, author of *The Joy of Sex*, and talking to men with 'sexual hang-ups' in an attempt to understand why Anderson had spurned her.

McKinney said: "They (the men) had said the sexual bondage game, where the woman was the aggressor, was the way to get over the guilt feelings of men who do not enjoy intercourse. When I came to England, I was looking for a real romantic cottage where we could have a honeymoon, and I decided to play some of those bondage games with him. We had such a fun time – just like old times."

Despite her protestations of innocence, Epsom magistrates decided she did have a case to answer. They committed her for a full Crown Court trial, but also granted her request to make a statement in court.

McKinney jumped at the chance and produced a fourteen-page document which covered her life story. In her strong southern drawl, she spoke of her conversion to Mormonism while studying at the Tennessee State University, her love affair with Anderson, her bizarre methods of satisfying his sexual guilt complex and, finally, how she became a Mormon outcast.

Her statement ended: "This man has imprisoned my heart with false promises of love and marriage and a family life. He has had me cast into prison for a kidnap he knows he set things up for. I don't want anything more to do with Kirk. He does not know what eternal love is. All I ask is that you do not allow him to imprison me any longer. Let me pick up the pieces of my life."

The court agreed to bail on sureties put up by McKinney's mother and at last Joyce was free. She became an instant celebrity, being escorted to the finest restaurants by reporters and photographed wherever she went in London.

Behind the scenes, a hectic auction was going on as the press clamoured for the rights to sell her life story. The bidding, she advised, ought to start at £50,000.

It was a heady lifestyle for the girl from Avery County, North Carolina, and it could not last. The media wanted to keep the story hot but the forthcoming trial meant they were heavily constrained as to what they could print. Inevitably, they used the time to dig dirt and it was in Los Angeles – where in 1975 McKinney had been chasing Anderson – that they found it.

Joyce had needed to pay the private detectives she had hired to follow Kirk's movements. She took to posing for bondage magazines and then graduated to providing sexual services for, as she put it, an 'upper income clientele'.

One of her adverts in the Los Angeles Free Press read: "Fantasy Room. Your fantasy is her speciality! – S&M (sadomasochism), B&D (bondage and dominance), escort service, PR work, acting jobs, nude wrestling/modelling, erotic phone calls, dirty panties or pictures, TV charm schools fantasies etc." The ad closed with a PS – "Joey says: Ah love shy boys, dirty ol' men and sugah daddies!" The enterprise earned her around $50,000 dollars a year.

While McKinney was awaiting trial, a file of photographs showing her performing perverted sexual acts was obtained by a London newspaper. It sat on its exclusive – but as it turned out, Joyce was to provide an even bigger story. On the eve of her trial, she and Keith packed their fourteen suitcases, picked up their British passports (made out in false identities) and flew to Shannon airport in Ireland. From there, posing as deaf mutes, they flew to Canada and later slipped back across the US border.

McKinney stayed on the run for fifteen months before the FBI tracked her down in North Carolina. She was convicted of using false passports, given three years probation and fined. That, it seemed, was the end of her extraordinary story.

But there was an epilogue. In June 1984 McKinney was arrested in Salt Lake City and accused of disturbing the peace by 'shadowing' Kirk Anderson.

Anderson complained that she was following and photographing him. Joyce retorted that she was simply writing a book and wanted to know what he was doing with his life. The case was thrown out of court after her lawyer entered a plea of 'extremely not guilty'.

BILLIE JEAN KING

In US sporting culture, few games carry higher kudos than tennis. Pushy parents start their children young, exhorting them to be ever faster, stronger and more expert. Apart from the potential financial rewards, the game is seen as a way of making social contacts and opening doors.

So when in April 1981 the legendary women's star Billie Jean King received a lawsuit from her former lesbian lover, the resulting scandal sent shock-waves through middle class America. In a so-called enlightened world, Billie Jean found herself vilified by her fickle public.

The ex-lover in question was Marilyn Barnett, a 33-year-old woman who acted as Billie Jean's personal aide, secretary, cook and cleaner. She was claiming rights to the 37-year-old star's fabulous Malibu Beach house, which she insisted Mrs King had promised her during the affair. She also demanded a lifetime's financial maintenance.

Marilyn claimed she had been 'secretary, confidante, companion, cook, cleaning person - all the things necessary to allow Mrs King to concentrate on her game'. Besieged by newspapermen, she then revealed why she was confined to a wheelchair. She had attempted suicide on learning of Billie Jean's intention to end

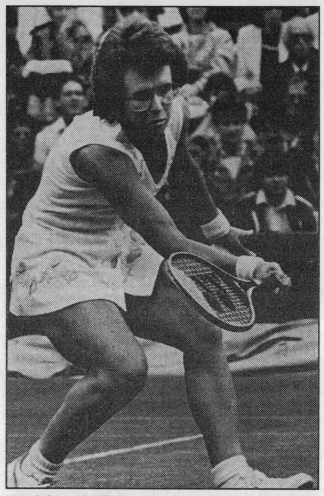

Tennis legend Billie Jean King was denounced by her lesbian lover.

the affair. Her 40 foot jump from an upstairs window at the disputed Malibu Beach property left her with a broken back.

At first Billie Jean denied the allegations as 'untrue and completely unfounded'. But two days later she called a press conference at which she admitted the lesbian affair with Barnett. In an emotionally-charged statement, she told journalists:

"It's been over for some time. I have always been honest and I have decided to talk to you as I have always talked to you – from the heart.

"I'm very disappointed and shocked that Marilyn has done this not only to herself – a very self-destructive thing – but also to other people who care for her. I now know who my friends are."

Those friends would be important to her. Billie Jean was about to enter the toughest battle of her life – as physically and emotionally draining as any of her twenty Wimbledon title wins. She had never denied the pleasure she obtained from sleeping with Marilyn and she was well aware how the affair would be viewed by the crusty, image-obsessed officials who ran the world game.

Days after the press conference she offered to resign as president of the Women's Tennis Association.

Already, big sports equipment firms were busy

cancelling the sponsorship contracts they had once so eagerly signed with her. They feared their own public image could be badly damaged.

The first part of the lawsuit opened in December 1981 and Billie Jean faced it with her loyal husband Larry at her side. The court had to decide whether Marilyn should be evicted from the Malibu Beach house and a decision was reached inside two days. The judge said Marilyn's claim 'bordered on extortion'. He dismissed it out of hand.

Outside court a jubilant Mrs King said: "The case has cost me millions of dollars in lost earnings from cancelled contracts. My fans have been absolutely wonderful. One thing I know is that Marilyn is not my friend. Larry and I have lost a lot."

Marilyn tried to be conciliatory and insisted that she still treasured the love letters Billie Jean had written during their seven-month relationship.

"I'm hostile towards Billie Jean," she said, "But I'll always love her. I hope the future holds good things for both of us."

Eleven months later Marilyn's claim for lifetime palimony was also rejected by a judge and Mrs King could at last put the scandal behind her. But before she did, she could not resist the temptation to set out her own feelings in her autobiography.

Pleading for more understanding from critics she wrote:

"Marilyn is small and blonde, with a little bird-like voice. She struck me as nice, easily affectionate and simple. What I liked most about her was that I could escape from everything. I felt no differently with Marilyn than when I was making love with a man. My point then was, as ever: 'Please, no labels.' "

CYNTHIA PAYNE

Whip-wielding Cynthia Payne – nick-named Madame Sin – was a brothel-keeper with a difference. Her ready smile and sense of humour meant that far from being vilified as a vice queen she became something of a folk legend in Britain. When she was finally hauled before a court in 1980, even the prosecution had to admit she managed 'a well-run brothel'.

Cynthia, then 46, ran a 'sex-for-luncheon-vouchers' establishment at her suburban house in Ambleside Avenue, Streatham, South London. Vicars, barristers, an MP and several peers counted themselves as regular customers. They would buy £25 worth of vouchers, which could then be traded in for the girls of their choice plus generous helpings of food and drink. When the police raided the house there were more than 50 men inside.

For each voucher the women, dubbed 'dedicated amateurs' by Cynthia, were paid a £6 fee. The atmosphere was more like a party for swingers than some seedy, sordid house of ill repute and reports of the sexual high-jinks were lapped up by a fascinated public. Later one of the regulars, a 74-year-old calling himself Squadron

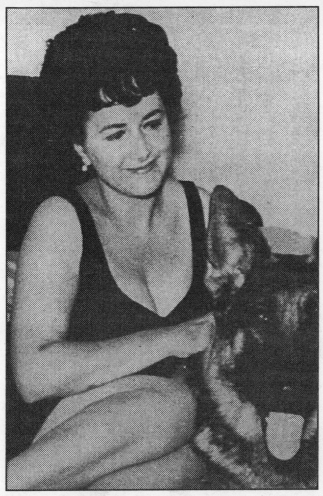

'Madame Sin': Cynthia Payne revelled in her
notorious nickname.

Leader Robert Smith, Retd., even gave guided tours.

Cynthia was sentenced to eighteen months on a charge of keeping a disorderly house, reduced on appeal to six months. She never expressed an ounce of regret for what she did and three years later told a reporter: "I'd like to think I'll be remembered for running a nice brothel, not one of those sordid places like they have in Soho. I should have been given the OBE for what I did for the country."

Her sexual philosophy was summed up by a large sign in her kitchen. It read:

"My House is CLEAN Enough To Be Healthy ... And DIRTY Enough To Be Happy."

MICHAEL TRESTRAIL

The security net cast around Queen Elizabeth II has, throughout her reign, grown ever tighter. Threats from terrorists, criminals, fame-seekers and the deranged have forced police constantly to re-assess the readiness and efficiency of the Royal Protection Squad. Senior officers have the unenviable problem of balancing security with the personal wishes and freedom of the Royal Family itself.

The embarrassment of failing to stop cockney Michael Fagan breaking in to Buckingham Palace was bad enough. That he was able to sit and chat with the Queen in her bedroom for ten minutes in June 1982 was almost beyond belief. Scotland Yard's hierarchy made loud mutterings about reviewing security and ensuring there would be no repeat scandal. Within a week of the *Daily Express* breaking the story of the Fagan affair, Yard commanders must have wished they'd chosen another career.

For among those who had read about Michael Fagan's exploits was a 38-year-old male prostitute called Michael Rauch, a Yorkshireman living in London. He believed he had an even bigger story to sell and he began touting it around Fleet Street with a price tag of £20,000. One newspaper began negotiations but then, realising the implications of what their informant was alleging, called in the police.

Rauch was questioned by detectives on 17 July 1982 and dropped his bombshell immediately. Did they know that Her Majesty's personal police bodyguard, Commander Michael Trestrail, was a promiscuous homosexual? And that he, Rauch, had been entertained by Trestrail inside Buckingham Palace itself.

At first it seemed hard to believe. Trestrail, 51, had passed a positive vetting check in the spring of 1982 and there was no reason to suspect that he led any kind of double life. But when confronted with the allegation he admitted it at once and offered his resignation, as it exposed one of the most important policemen in the country to blackmail. (Rauch had indeed tried and failed to blackmail Trestrail earlier in the year.)

Later the commander's solicitor David Napley issued a statement expressing his client's 'deep sorrow' for the embarrassment he had heaped on the Royal Family and Scotland Yard. He had a deep respect for both institutions "towards whose service his only objective had been to devote himself, including ensuring the safety of Her Majesty."

Now the media had its scalp, the finger of

blame was shifted towards those responsible for the positive vetting of Trestrail. But a Security Commission headed by Lord Bridge of Harwich later made clear that there should be no recriminations against the vetting officer responsible. Lord Bridge asserted: "If a man in a public position leads a secret double-life and succeeds, as Trestrail did for so long, in maintaining a total and effective separation between the two sides of his activities, this must present the positive vetting investigator with an almost impossible task."

The Commission ruled that none of the commander's numerous affairs had resulted in any danger to palace security. Lord Bridge went out of his way to point this out stressing: "Commander Trestrail carried out his duties as Queen's police officer loyally and efficiently, but led a secret double-life in that he indulged in promiscuous homosexual activities, mostly with prostitutes."

Although the officer had known he was a homosexual from his school days, he had tried to keep his sexuality secret. However, his feelings sometimes became overpowering; he would go out drinking with friends and would then procure prostitutes.

Lord Bridge pointed out: "In the result the occasions of his homosexual activity have been spasmodic and infrequent, separated by periods of months according to his own account ... there was no breach of security and, in my judgement, security was not put at risk."

The Bridge report went on to deliver a mild slap on the wrist to the police for failing to investigate information from an officer identified only as 'X'. This Mr 'X' had reported his belief that Trestrail was a practising homosexual to his superiors, shortly after the commander was given the Palace appointment. But the tip was ignored.

Lord Bridge revealed: "On hearing of Trestrail's resignation, 'X' very properly communicated with Scotland Yard, volunteered a statement and in due course gave evidence before me. The substance ... was that twice after Trestrail's joining the Royal Protection Group, 'X' reported to Commander Perkins, who was then the Queen's Police Officer, that Trestrail was a homosexual. According to 'X', Commander Perkins simply brushed the matter aside, telling 'X', in effect, that it was nothing to do with him."

By the time of the Commission's investigation, Commander Perkins had died. Lord Bridge observed that while 'X' was a loyal and genuine witness he had been unable to present Perkins with a single hard fact to back his allegation.

Trestrail's decision to resign was endorsed by the inquiry as the only acceptable choice.

"Doubts as to the soundness of his judgement," it observed, "and public opinion with regard to indiscriminate promiscuity would, in any case, have made it impossible for him to continue."

The two leading characters in the Trestrail affair became poles apart in its aftermath. Trestrail continued to lead a comfortable life and, despite cruel gossip about his lump-sum pay-off of £25,000 and his £600-per-month pension, he eased himself back into the Establishment's favour. Rauch was later found dead and bereft of any money at his flat in Notting Hill Gate.

An unidentified friend later said of him: "No one wanted to know him because he had betrayed Michael Trestrail and embarrassed the Queen. The gay community loathed him."

CECIL PARKINSON

In the summer of 1983 Cecil Parkinson enjoyed a status close to hero worship among the British Conservative Party faithful. His charm and good looks had long won him an army of female admirers among the blue rinse set in the constituencies. His background in industry had earned him the respect of the party's principal business backers. And his calm, assured performance for the cameras at the height of the Falklands War the previous year had marked him down as a possible future prime minister.

When, as party chairman, Parkinson delivered a landslide victory for Margaret Thatcher in the general election of 9 June 1983 it seemed almost everything he touched turned to gold. Millions of TV viewers watched him at her side, waving from an upstairs window at Conservative Central Office as he triumphantly acknowledged the cheering crowds below.

From his beaming smile, no one could have guessed at the inner torment plagueing him. In fact Cecil Parkinson was fighting to keep the lid on the biggest political sex scandal since Lord Lambton's dalliance with a callgirl ten years earlier.

As the lights burned into the small hours at the

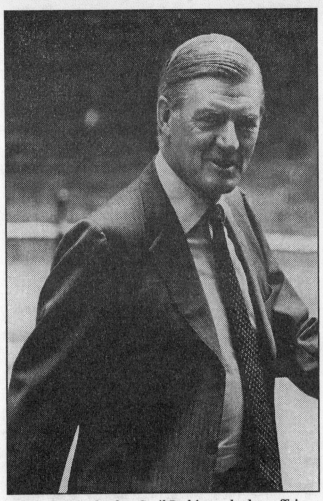

Political powerbroker Cecil Parkinson had an affair with his secretary.

London HQ of the Tory party, the dilemma Parkinson faced was agonising. Should he marry his pregnant mistress and former constituency secretary, Sarah Keays? Or should he opt to stick with his wife Ann and try to put the affair behind him?

According to Miss Keays, Parkinson had twice promised to marry her and twice changed his mind. The first time was in 1979 – the year Mrs Thatcher swept to power – when he offered to leave his family and seek a divorce. But the pledge came to nothing and Parkinson, by now a junior transport minister, stayed with his wife.

The second time, Miss Keays claims, was the June 1983 polling day itself, some months after their affair had been re-kindled. Only a few weeks earlier she had told him she was pregnant with their child and he had replied that he would not marry her and would not inform Mrs Thatcher of his personal difficulties. Now he had changed his mind again. She claimed he proposed and called Downing Street soon afterwards to explain his decision.

The prospect of a marriage split, and the inevitable tidal wave of publicity that would follow, must have filled 52-year-old Parkinson with dread. Up until now his life and career had been the very model of respectability: a scholarship to Cambridge, then management experience with the Metal Box Company and later a plum job with a respected City firm of accountants.

His political career, too, had been on an upward spiral from the moment he entered the House of Commons as MP for Enfield West in 1970. Within four years he was a junior whip in the administration of Premier Edward Heath and later served as Opposition spokesman on trade. Under Mrs Thatcher, he was quickly promoted to Paymaster General and party chairman, an obvious sign that she regarded his loyalty and sensitive political antennae as vital to the Tories' future prospects. The railwayman's son from Carnforth, Lancashire, was consequently regarded by his colleagues as a safe pair of hands.

In August 1983 Parkinson, now Trade and Industry Secretary, took his family abroad on holiday. Miss Keays later insisted that she believed he still intended to marry her. She had good reason to hope he would break the news to his wife quickly because Westminster was fast becoming rife with gossip. On 23 August journalists from the *Daily Mirror* had called at her house and asked directly if she was expecting a baby by the Trade Secretary.

On 1 September she met Parkinson, at his request, in a London office. There he dropped his bombshell, telling her that while abroad he had decided he would not and could not marry her. The stage was set for a public scandal and it was not long coming.

Within a few days the magazine *Private Eye* published a paragraph referring to Parkinson's 'marital difficulties' and mentioning Miss Keays's pregnancy. Realising he could not allow the matter to drift, Parkinson decided to come clean before he could be exposed. He issued a statement through his solicitors which ran:

"...I have had a relationship with Miss Keays for a number of years. During our relationship I told Miss Keays of my wish to marry her. Despite my having given Miss Keays that assurance, my wife, who has been a great source of strength, and I decided to stay together to keep our family together."

Soon afterwards Mrs Thatcher gave her personal endorsement in a statement from Downing Street which included the phrase: "Resignation does not... and will not arise."

The affair exploded just as the Tory party was gathering in Blackpool for its annual conference in October 1983. In the bars and restaurants delegates talked of little else. Could Parkinson survive? What other revelations could be expected? They didn't have long to wait.

Perhaps realising that his career was on the line, Parkinson agreed to appear on the BBC's flagship current affairs programme *Panorama*. There he defended his actions, expressed his regret at the way things had turned out and insisted that the Prime Minister had been kept fully informed. He also suggested that the full facts behind the affair had been set out in his earlier statement.

It was this insistence that drove the final nail into his political coffin. Sarah Keays saw things differently. And while Parkinson was an accomplished politician and public speaker, his mistress, daughter of a colonel, proved a more than worthy adversary.

In a statement through her solicitors, she said Parkinson had implied that she tried to trap him into marriage; further, that she had tried to destroy his reputation and had prevented the matter from being kept quiet. The final accusation, she said, "presumes that I should hide from public view and declare on the baby's birth certificate 'father unknown', so casting further doubt on my reputation and denying the child his fundamental right to know the identity of his father."

The truth, according to Miss Keays, was very different. Far from trying to trap the minister, she had conceived their child as part of a loving and long-standing relationship which she believed would end in marriage. She had accepted his decision not to marry her but made clear her baby would grow up knowing the identity of its father. She had hoped a joint statement from their respective solicitors would forestall any press 'scoop'. Miss Keays continued:

"On Wednesday, October 5, when I was informed of what had been published in *Private Eye*, I telephoned Mr Parkinson and told him that if he did not issue the statement which solicitors had been discussing for some weeks, then I would be obliged to defend myself."

"Press comment, government pronouncements, and the continued speculation about this matter have placed me in an impossible position. I feel that I have both a public duty and a duty to my family to put the record straight."

The text of the statement was issued to *The Times* on 13 October 1983 – the penultimate day of the conference. As soon as the newspaper's first edition dropped in Downing Street a copy of the statement was faxed to Mrs Thatcher's Blackpool hotel room. At 2am Cecil Parkinson briefly met the Prime Minister in her suite before returning to his wife Ann, waiting in their own room, to decide his future. A mere six hours later he again knocked on Mrs Thatcher's door and asked her to accept his resignation from the Cabinet.

It was a shattering blow, but it was not the end

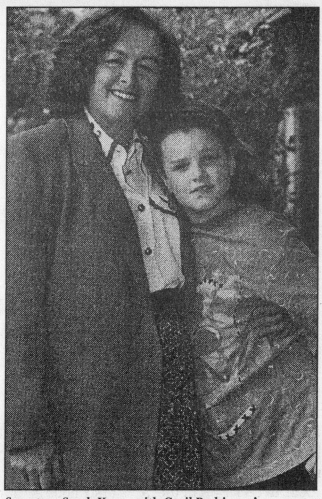

Secretary Sarah Keays with Cecil Parkinson's love child.

of his career. After four years in the political wilderness he was brought back into the Cabinet as Mrs Thatcher's Energy Secretary. When news leaked out, reporters besieged the Parkinson's country home north of London to rake over the Keays' affair. Typically, Parkinson met them with his usual mixture of charm and gravitas. The journalists and photographers were invited into the back garden for coffee. Though his affair with Sara Keays' cropped up several times, the new minister never breathed her name. To the watching world he and Ann were clearly united once more.

After his spell as Energy Secretary, Parkinson went on to head the Department of Transport. But he recognised that his political future had been fatally flawed by the Keays affair. In 1990 he returned to the Commons backbenches and quit his seat at the 1992 election to join the House of Lords as a life peer.

JIMMY SWAGGART

Jimmy Swaggart was a braggart. The television evangelist boasted that he was incorruptible, unlike his rival preacher, Jim Bakker. Most of his flock believed him – until they heard what he got up to in a seedy New Orleans motel room.

Prostitute Debra Murphee was regularly employed by Swaggart to perform obscene sex acts while he watched from the comfort of an armchair. Murphee went along with the lucrative sex games until the preacher suggested that she invite her nine-year-old daughter to watch also.

The mother, who had a record for prostitution offences in two sates, said she was so disgusted that she went public with her story. She recreated Swaggart's favourite poses for Penthouse magazine, and the sixteen pages of explicit pictures were deemed so hot that they had to be sealed in each issue. Murphee also went on a national media tour to publicise her revelations.

Swaggart also went on national television and tearfully confessed to 'a moral sin', although he did not specify what it was.

The Louisiana Assemblies of God were inclined to deal with him leniently; they recommended a three-month suspension from preaching. The national church ordered Swaggart banished from the pulpit for a full year, and the state organisation reluctantly adopted that punishment. Swaggart, however, unwisely defied the ban after only a few months on the grounds that his absence would destroy his $140 million-a-year worldwide ministries. He was immediately defrocked by the Assemblies Of God.

Murphee faded from the scene after a proposed movie deal about her meetings with the dirty preacher failed to come to fruition. Swaggart, meanwhile, saw his television empire dwindle from tens of millions of viewers to mere thousands. He tells his congregation that the Lord has forgiven him for his sins, adding piously: "What's past is past."

BISHOP CASEY

As Ireland's Bishop of Galway, Eamonn Casey knew only too well the rules the Catholic Church laid down about the sex lives of its priests.

Strictest among these was the demand for celibacy; a huge personal sacrifice yet one considered sacrosanct to the cherished traditions and public perception of the Church.

So when in 1973 the 46-year-old Casey, then Bishop of Kerry, indulged in a passionate affair with a telephonist, Annie Murphy, he knew the potential consequences of his lust. The effect on his personal relationship with his God was something he could work on privately. The effect on his career as a churchman could be a highly embarrassing scandal capable of destroying him.

Casey's affair with Murphy, which blossomed in 1973, ended with the birth of his son, Peter, in a Dublin hospital in July of the following year. Annie, frightened of the implications, took her baby out of the country soon afterwards to stay with close family in New York. But by the time he was six months old she had returned, keen to discuss the way Peter's future would be handled. She knew enough about Catholicism to realise the talks would be conducted in absolute secrecy.

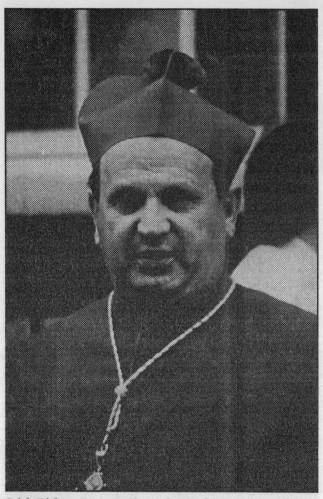

Irish Bishop Eamonn Casey broke his solemn oath of celibacy.

At that first meeting Casey brought along a junior priest, perhaps to ensure that emotions would necessarily be restrained. He clutched Murphy's hand with a whispered greeting but his glance warned her that they should not appear too familiar. Though he smiled and cuddled his son like any father, the impression given was that he was merely welcoming an old friend and her family back to Ireland.

That re-union set the pattern for the months ahead. Casey welcomed any opportunity to see the boy. But he showed no inclination to formalise his new parental role with any kind of public recognition; not even with the guaranteed confidentiality of a maintenance agreement.

Gradually, Annie realised that she was in grave danger of mishandling her future. If she stayed in Ireland, Peter would inevitably grow closer to his father but with no hope of obtaining his birthright. As the months turned into years, she feared, so it would become harder and harder to leave.

By early 1975 Annie and Peter were back in New York. She had opened negotiations for maintenance payments, to which he responded with an offer of $50 per month. This was later increased to $300 per quarter. Finally, as talks between them grew ever more acrimonious, Casey made a 'final offer' of $175 per month.

For the next few years contact between the parents was minimal. But Annie didn't lose track of Eamonn. She could hardly fail to notice his high profile campaign against the Reagan administration over its aid for right-wing forces in El Salvador. Casey had urged his own government to break off diplomatic relations with the US, a naive hope considering the number of American dollars that benevolent Irish-Americans invest in the old country. He also condemned Dublin's 'callous' attitude to the Third World and attacked senior politicians for making minute aid contributions.

In her book *The True Story of my Secret Love for the Bishop of Galway: Forbidden Fruit* Annie recalls: "In view of Eamonn's tiny payment to us, I was amused by his stout defence of the poor."

"I had spent four months writing to him. With the cost of living rising it was vital to get him to contribute more to his son's upbringing. After he had refused several times I called him. 'Listen carefully Eamonn, because I am not repeating this. My lawyer is hungry. He'd love to take you to court over maintenance. So it's either $275 a month or your neck.'"

From now on Casey's hopes of covering up the scandal were doomed. He knew it too. When Annie's Scots-born boyfriend Arthur Pennell confronted him in his study at Galway, Casey played a cat-and-mouse game in which he denied all knowledge of a son. Asked about the maintenance payments he had already made he replied: "Prove it!" According to Annie he claimed he would "resign rather than have anything to do with her boy."

By 1990, Annie and Peter had hit rock bottom. Their money had all but run out and they were living a hand to mouth existence in cheap motels as they drove west across America in search of a new life. They had been swamped with court orders, injunctions and loan-settlement demands. Annie decided the time for informal arrangements was over. She went to see a top New York attorney, Peter McKay. Immediately, he began seeking personal damages for her with instructions to settle for not less than a $100,000 lump sum settlement.

In the end, Casey settled for a total payment of $125,000 dollars. He also asked that Peter sign a document relinquishing all future rights to any paternity claim. McKay rejected the proposal out of hand.

During talks with the lawyer, Casey had his first face-to-face meeting with Peter in years. According to the boy, Casey asked him what he hoped to do with his life and told him he prayed for him twice a day. Then it was goodbye. Their time together was barely four minutes.

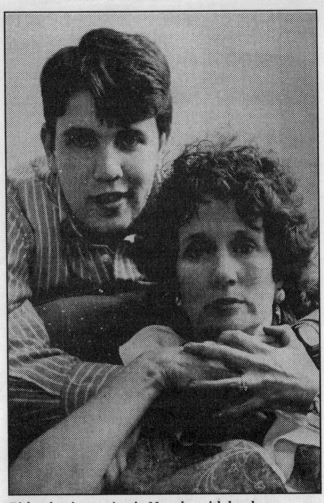

Bishop's mistress Annie Murphy with her love child Peter.

Embittered by this reaction, and Casey's refusal to recognise his own son publicly, Peter and his mother resolved to raise the stakes. When some months later the Bishop called Annie to say he would again be visiting New York, she arranged to see him in the lobby of the Hyatt Hotel. She planned to be wired for sound and to persuade a friend, Jim Powers, to record every second of the meeting on a camcorder.

Annie later recalled how she felt a surprising sense of tenderness when she set eyes on her former lover. He kissed and hugged her and stroked her face. She suggested spending the night together to talk, and then tearfully left him for a few minutes to visit the ladies washroom. On the way back Peter, who had been hiding behind a potted plant, told her that the filming and recording had been a success. Annie returned to Casey and told him: "Peter's here."

"Good."

"You mean you'll see him?"

"No, he can take you home."

"Too late, he's just gone. Besides, I told Peter I was spending the night with you."

"God Almighty. You told your son ..."

"Our son."

"... that you are spending the night with a bishop?"

"He does realise that I did it before."

The following day Peter resolved to begin a legal fight to extract maintenance arrears and a contribution towards his education costs. But the lawyers he contacted would not take on the case. Instead they advised an 'unofficial' agreement. Faced with this obstacle, Peter decided the time had come to end offers of what he called 'dirt money' and blow the whole scandal open.

In early May 1992 Arthur Pennell rang *The Irish Times* on behalf of Annie and Peter to offer a world exclusive story. He also called Casey and told him what they planned. Casey pleaded with them not to betray him.

Yet even as a team of reporters began checking the secret sex life of the Bishop of Galway, the target of their investigation had decided enough was enough. He resigned, admitting that he had taken around £70,000 from Irish Church funds to help meet the maintenance and damages payments to Annie. That money, he said, had since been re-paid by a friend. He refused to confirm rumours that the benefactor in question was none other than Senator Edward Kennedy.

The scandal sent instant shock waves through the Catholic Church, particularly its Irish hierarchy. There were few apologists for the Bishop; most agreed he got what he deserved.

Casey fled first to New York and then to San Antonio, Texas, where he took refuge in the

Mother House of the Sisters of Charity Incarnate. He remained there until March 1993 when he decamped to a new retreat run by the Sisters in Cuernavaca, south of Mexico City. There he was known to most of the nuns only as Padre Sean.

The following month, Casey gave an interview to *The Sunday Express* in which he rejected many of the claims made in Annie Murphy's book. He also suggested she had had another 'fling' with a man during his own affair with her.

Asked about sexual encounters in the back of his car, or on a rug to the songs of Frank Sinatra, he replied: "The memories left in my mouth are a very different taste."

He went on: "Why did she do it? For money? For some kind of revenge on the Church. On me? For what?"

Then he stalked back to the privacy of his exile, where he could ponder the answer in peace.

GARY HART

Senator Gary Hart finally lost his chance to become President of the United States of America when he tried to prove that he was an honest man! His reputation as a womaniser was so strong that the campaigner for the Democratic nomination took the extraordinarily daring step of challenging the media to follow him – thus supposedly proving that he was a clean-living family man and hard-working politician.

The Miami Herald accepted the challenge. They followed him throughout a weekend in which he romped with a leggy blonde named Donna Rice. It transpired that Hart had been seeing Rice for months – and had even been on a sailing jaunt round the Caribbean on a yacht aptly named *Monkey Business*.

Gary Hart denied that anything untoward had taken place. His loyal wife, Lee, stood staunchly by him. But the public did not fall for this show of moral rectitude. And shortly afterwards evidence arose of two previous liaisons which he admitted took place during separations from Lee in 1979 and 1981.

Hart admitted the affairs with English 'professional hostess' Diana Phillips and with

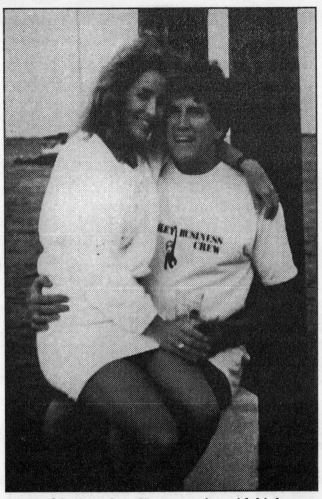

Sex-mad Senator Gary Hart cavorting with his lover Donna Rice.

Iowa political aide Lynn Carter. However, he sidestepped questions about a third lady friend, Marilyn Youngbird, described by a magazine as a 'radiant divorcee' and by Hart himself as his 'spiritual adviser'. Youngbird, an American Indian, revealed that she and Hart took part in a Comanche ceremony during which 'we brushed the front and back of our bodies with eagle feathers'. It was, added Miss Youngbird, 'very sensual'.

After the revelations, the Democratic hopeful retired to private life. Meanwhile, the cause of his downfall, Donna Rice, was bombarded with offers to kiss and tell. Instead, she took up acting studies at a tiny community theatre in Virginia where, according to a friend, she also 'does volunteer work, helping the disabled and the terminally ill. She just wants her privacy'.

MIKE TYSON

World heavyweight boxing champion Mike Tyson easily ranked among the sport's all-time greats. But his carefully-crafted image as a great athlete was destroyed forever in 1991 after he raped eighteen-year-old beauty contestant Desiree Washington. Tyson was convicted and jailed for six years.

It was the ultimate low point in a personal life that had turned into a shambles. He had developed a habit for anti-depressant drugs and was drinking copious amounts of cheap rum. He was also relatively broke. Over the years dozens of middle men had creamed off 95 cents from each of the hundreds of million dollars he generated.

The highly-public collapse of Tyson's marriage to actress Robin Givens in 1989 had been a devastating humiliation. She called him a "mental case" on national television and described her life with him as "pure hell". She told another interviewer:

"Mike should be required to wear a sign that says 'Caution, Mike Tyson is hazardous to women.' He's a demon underneath. He's got a terrible temper. I was terrified of him."

Those words came back to haunt Tyson at his trial. The jury heard how in July 1991 he had met Desiree, from Coventry, Rhode Island, at the Indiana Black Expo celebrations in Indianapolis. He promised to take her on a round of parties at which she would meet many of her celebrity heroes. But after picking her up he invited her to his hotel room on the pretext of making a couple of telephone calls. Then he raped her.

At his trial Tyson was found guilty and sentenced to six years in prison. When he later tried to get his prison term reduced the trial judge bluntly told him his actions were 'disgraceful' and upheld the original sentence.

In June 1994 Tyson repeated his claims of innocence and said he had begun a new life under the guidance of Islam. He told an American magazine: "I know that I did bad things. I know I treated people, women badly, but all that is behind me. Whatever they say, I never raped that girl. I will never admit to doing that. I will go to my grave knowing that I didn't do that. I am sorry for all the pain it has caused to her and her family."